Nutrition Book For Women

Crafted by Skriuwer

Copyright © 2024 by Skriuwer.

All rights reserved. No part of this book may be used or reproduced in any form whatsoever without written permission except in the case of brief quotations in critical articles or reviews.

For more information, contact : **kontakt@skriuwer.com** (www.skriuwer.com)

TABLE OF CONTENTS

CHAPTER 1: INTRODUCTION

- Why women's nutrition is uniquely important
- Overview of key health concerns and how to address them
- Myths and misunderstandings in women's nutrition

CHAPTER 2: UNDERSTANDING NUTRITION BASICS

- Defining calories and how they impact energy balance
- Overview of macronutrients (carbs, proteins, fats)
- Basics of micronutrients and hydration

CHAPTER 3: NUTRIENTS FOR WOMEN'S HEALTH

- Essential nutrients supporting female body functions
- Fiber, antioxidants, and their benefits
- Practical tips for boosting nutrient intake

CHAPTER 4: VITAMINS, MINERALS, AND OTHER MICRONUTRIENTS

- Detailed look at vitamins A to K
- Critical minerals like iron, calcium, magnesium
- Recognizing and addressing micronutrient gaps

CHAPTER 5: HORMONES AND HOW THEY AFFECT NUTRITION

- Hormonal fluctuations in different life stages
- Impact on appetite, weight, and mood
- Strategies to balance food choices and hormone changes

CHAPTER 6: REPRODUCTIVE HEALTH AND NUTRITION

- Supporting menstrual health and fertility
- Addressing conditions like PCOS and endometriosis
- Nutrition for a healthy menstrual cycle

CHAPTER 7: NUTRITION THROUGH DIFFERENT LIFE STAGES

- Unique needs during adolescence, adulthood, and seniors
- Bone health, muscle maintenance, and energy demands
- Adjusting diet to ever-changing body requirements

CHAPTER 8: HEALTHY EATING PATTERNS AND MEAL PLANNING

- Creating balanced meals that fit your lifestyle
- Meal-prepping techniques for busy schedules
- Portion control and mindful eating tips

CHAPTER 9: SPECIAL DIETS AND FOOD CHOICES

- Vegetarian, vegan, gluten-free, and other dietary approaches
- Pros and cons of low-carb, keto, paleo diets
- Personalizing diets for health and preference

CHAPTER 10: MANAGING WEIGHT IN A HEALTHY WAY

- Calorie balance and portion control principles
- Avoiding crash diets and embracing steady progress
- Combining nutrition with exercise for sustainable results

CHAPTER 11: ENERGY, PERFORMANCE, AND EXERCISE

- *Fueling your body for workouts and daily activity*
- *Pre- and post-workout nutrition*
- *Hydration and recovery essentials*

CHAPTER 12: EMOTIONAL EATING AND BODY IMAGE

- *Recognizing and managing emotional triggers*
- *Developing a positive relationship with food*
- *Strategies to improve body image and self-esteem*

CHAPTER 13: ADDRESSING COMMON NUTRITIONAL DEFICIENCIES

- *Iron, vitamin D, calcium, B12, and other key gaps*
- *Symptoms, causes, and practical solutions*
- *Preventing deficiencies through diet and supplements*

CHAPTER 14: PREGNANCY AND POSTPARTUM NUTRITION

- *Nutrient needs before, during, and after pregnancy*
- *Managing morning sickness, cravings, and postpartum recovery*
- *Breastfeeding support and healthy weight considerations*

CHAPTER 15: MENOPAUSE AND BEYOND

- *Hormonal changes and bone health*
- *Managing hot flashes, mood swings, and weight fluctuations*
- *Nutritional focus for long-term vitality*

CHAPTER 16: BOOSTING IMMUNITY THROUGH FOOD

- *Key vitamins, minerals, and antioxidants for defense*
- *Gut health, probiotics, and reducing inflammation*
- *Lifestyle habits that strengthen immune response*

CHAPTER 17: BUILDING HEALTHY HABITS AND SETTING GOALS

- *Why small, consistent actions lead to lasting change*
- *SMART goal-setting and habit-stacking methods*
- *Tracking progress and staying motivated*

CHAPTER 18: OVERCOMING CHALLENGES AND BARRIERS

- *Time, budget, and emotional obstacles to healthy living*
- *Social pressures, family dynamics, and limited access to foods*
- *Adapting strategies for real-world success*

CHAPTER 19: SELF-CARE, MINDSET, AND STRESS MANAGEMENT

- *Connecting mental well-being with nutritional choices*
- *Daily practices for relaxation and positive thinking*
- *Building resilience through self-care routines*

CHAPTER 20: BRINGING IT ALL TOGETHER AND LONG-TERM SUCCESS

- *Summarizing key lessons for women's nutrition*
- *Staying flexible through different life stages*
- *Maintaining balance, adaptability, and a positive mindset*

CHAPTER 1: INTRODUCTION

1.1 Why Nutrition Matters for Women

Nutrition matters for everyone, but for women, it is especially important. Women's bodies go through many changes throughout life. These changes involve hormonal shifts, pregnancy, menopause, and other factors that affect the body's needs. Having enough of the right foods can help manage these changes, keep energy levels steady, and lower the risk of health problems. Good nutrition also helps women feel stronger and more confident in daily life.

Many women juggle multiple roles. They might work outside the home, care for children, or take on many other responsibilities. With so many demands, nutrition can sometimes be overlooked. Skipping meals, eating junk food on the run, or ignoring personal health can happen when you are busy. This book aims to make nutrition simple so that women of all backgrounds can understand why healthy eating is important and how to make it work in a busy life.

1.2 Common Health Concerns for Women

Women may have health concerns that are different from men. Some of these are tied to hormone levels. Others are linked to lifestyle or genetics. Examples of common health concerns include:

- **Bone health**: Women tend to have a higher risk of osteoporosis. This is a condition where bones become weak and can break easily.
- **Iron deficiency**: Due to monthly blood loss through menstruation, many women have low iron levels, which can lead to fatigue and weakness.
- **Pregnancy-related issues**: If a woman becomes pregnant, she needs extra nutrients like folic acid, iron, and calcium to help the baby grow and keep her own body healthy.

- **Menopause**: When women reach menopause, hormone levels change. This can affect bone health, weight, mood, and other areas.

The good news is that many of these concerns can be managed or even prevented by making thoughtful food choices. Understanding which foods provide the most benefit and how to balance meals can lead to better overall health.

1.3 The Purpose and Approach of This Book

Nutrition Book for Women: A Guide to Optimal Health and Well-being was written with one goal in mind: to make it easy to learn about nutrition. The chapters will guide you step by step. This book uses basic English so that most readers, including younger ones, can understand it. If there is a scientific term, it will be explained in simple words.

Another goal is to show you that healthy eating is not about perfection. It is about balance and forming habits that are realistic for your own life. Everyone's life is different, so there is no one-size-fits-all plan. Instead, you will find guidelines, advice, and tips to help you create a plan that fits you.

1.4 What You Can Expect to Learn

1. **Basic Nutrition**: You will learn about the building blocks of food—carbohydrates, proteins, and fats—and understand the role of vitamins and minerals.
2. **How the Female Body Works**: We will look at how hormones can affect your appetite, energy levels, and even your mood.
3. **Healthy Eating Patterns**: We will discuss ways to plan meals and snacks that keep you feeling full and satisfied.
4. **Nutrition Through Life Stages**: From teenage years to pregnancy to menopause, your nutritional needs can change. We will outline how to meet those needs.

5. **Building Positive Habits**: You will find practical advice on how to form healthy habits and overcome common barriers like lack of time or limited budget.

1.5 Why Simplicity Matters

It is easy to feel overwhelmed by nutrition. There are countless diets, trends, and news stories. Some say carbs are bad; others say fats are worse. Sometimes, it feels like you need a nutrition degree just to pick the right foods. This book takes a simpler approach. By focusing on balanced eating and basic principles, you can avoid confusion and focus on practical steps. The goal is to provide clear, direct information so you can decide what is right for you.

1.6 Myths and Misunderstandings in Women's Nutrition

Before we dive deep, let's address some myths:

1. **Myth: Women need fewer calories than men, always.**
   While it is true that on average, men have more muscle mass and may burn more calories, each person is unique. A very active woman might need more calories than a less active man. It depends on body composition, lifestyle, and health goals.
2. **Myth: Low-fat diets are always healthiest.**
   The truth is that certain fats (like those from avocados, nuts, and seeds) are good for you. A low-fat diet might leave out these good fats and might not benefit your health in the long run.
3. **Myth: Carbs are the enemy.**
   Complex carbohydrates from whole grains, beans, and vegetables are important for energy. Not all carbs are bad. It is refined carbs and sugary snacks that often cause problems.
4. **Myth: Women cannot build muscle.**
   Women can build muscle, but at a different rate than men

because of hormone differences. Protein and strength training can still help women develop lean muscle.
5. **Myth: Supplements can replace a healthy diet.** Supplements can be helpful if you have a deficiency, but they do not replace real food. Whole foods contain nutrients, fiber, and other substances that supplements cannot fully provide.

1.7 A Look at What Lies Ahead

- **Chapter 2** will give you a foundation in nutrition basics—calories, proteins, carbs, fats, and how they interact in the body.
- After that, we will tackle topics such as vitamins, minerals, hormones, and the specific nutritional needs of women at different ages.
- There will be sections on emotional eating, body image, and how to handle diet-related stress.
- We will also talk about the specific changes that happen during pregnancy, postpartum, and menopause.
- Lastly, we will discuss how to create a long-term plan that includes not only food but also self-care and mindset.

1.8 How to Use This Book

Feel free to read it cover to cover or jump to sections that interest you. Each chapter stands on its own but also connects to the overall theme of balanced, healthy living. We have avoided repeating the same content in different chapters so that each topic is fresh, yet ties into the bigger picture.

1.9 The Importance of Balance Over Perfection

A key theme in this book is that trying to be "perfect" can create stress, which can sabotage healthy habits. Aim for balance instead. Some days, you might eat more sweets than you planned. Other days, you might eat a big salad for lunch and skip dessert. Over time, it is your overall pattern that matters. Avoid blaming yourself for small missteps. The important thing is to keep moving forward.

1.10 Setting Realistic Goals

If you want to lose weight, gain muscle, or just feel better overall, set small goals. For example, start by adding an extra serving of vegetables each day. Once you do that consistently, focus on replacing sugary drinks with water or herbal tea. By making small but steady changes, you create habits that last. Crash diets or drastic changes often lead to burnout or weight regain.

1.11 The Mind-Body Connection

Women often experience strong connections between emotions and food. Stress, hormones, and life events can make it easy to use food as comfort. Being aware of this connection can help you make healthier choices and manage stress in ways that do not involve harmful eating habits.

1.12 Stories and Examples

Throughout the chapters, you will find examples of how women can handle challenges—like balancing nutrition and a busy work schedule, or cooking meals for a family while also meeting your personal goals. These examples are meant to show that many of us share similar struggles, and there are ways to overcome them.

CHAPTER 2: UNDERSTANDING NUTRITION BASICS

2.1 What Is Nutrition?

Nutrition is the study of how the body uses food. We eat foods that contain various nutrients. These nutrients have different roles: they may provide energy, help build tissues, or support body processes. Good nutrition means getting enough of each nutrient without going overboard on unhealthy ones.

2.2 Why Calories Matter

A **calorie** is a measure of energy. When we talk about calories in food, we're talking about the potential energy the body can use to function. If you eat more calories than your body needs, it might store them as fat. If you eat fewer, your body might break down stored fat or muscle to compensate. The number of calories a person needs depends on factors like age, height, weight, activity level, and metabolism.

- **Basal Metabolic Rate (BMR)**: This is the number of calories your body needs at rest just to keep you alive (breathing, circulating blood, etc.).
- **Physical Activity**: Exercise and daily tasks increase how many calories you burn.
- **Thermic Effect of Food**: The body uses energy to digest, absorb, and process the food you eat.

2.3 Macronutrients: Carbohydrates, Proteins, and Fats

There are three main nutrients that provide calories (energy). They are called **macronutrients** because you need them in relatively large amounts. Each one has a specific job in the body.

2.3.1 Carbohydrates

- **Role**: Carbs are the body's main source of energy.
- **Types**:
    1. **Simple Carbohydrates (Sugars)**: Found in fruits, milk, table sugar, and sweets. They provide quick energy but can also lead to fast spikes in blood sugar.
    2. **Complex Carbohydrates**: Found in whole grains, legumes, vegetables, and other unprocessed plant foods. They provide slower, more sustained energy.
- **Daily Need**: The exact amount varies. Most guidelines suggest that around 45–65% of daily calories come from carbohydrates, especially those from whole foods.
- **Fiber**: A special type of carbohydrate that is not fully digested but helps with bowel regularity, blood sugar control, and satiety (the feeling of fullness).

2.3.2 Proteins

- **Role**: Protein builds and repairs tissues, makes enzymes and hormones, and supports immune function.
- **Sources**: Lean meats, fish, poultry, eggs, dairy, beans, lentils, nuts, and seeds.
- **Daily Need**: Often recommended 10–35% of daily calories from protein. A common guideline is about 0.8 grams of protein per kilogram of body weight for the average adult. But needs can be higher for pregnant women, athletes, or older adults.
- **Complete vs. Incomplete Proteins**:
    - **Complete proteins** have all the essential amino acids your body needs and are found mostly in animal foods.
    - **Incomplete proteins** lack one or more essential amino acids and are often found in plant foods. By mixing different plant sources (like beans and rice), you can get complete protein.

2.3.3 Fats

- **Role**: Fats provide a concentrated source of energy, help absorb vitamins, support cell growth, and make hormones.
- **Types**:
    1. **Unsaturated Fats**: Found in nuts, seeds, avocados, and fish. Often called "good fats."
    2. **Saturated Fats**: Found in high amounts in red meat, butter, and cheese. It's recommended to limit these.
    3. **Trans Fats**: Often found in processed foods, pastries, and some margarines. These are considered harmful and should be avoided whenever possible.
- **Daily Need**: It is generally recommended to keep total fat intake around 20–35% of daily calories, focusing on unsaturated fats over saturated or trans fats.

2.4 Micronutrients: Vitamins and Minerals

In later chapters, we will explore these in detail. For now, understand that vitamins and minerals do not provide calories, but they help the body function properly. Some vitamins (A, D, E, and K) are fat-soluble, meaning they need fat to be absorbed. Others are water-soluble (B vitamins and vitamin C).

Minerals like calcium, iron, and magnesium are needed for various processes such as bone formation, oxygen transport, and muscle function.

2.5 Water: The Often Overlooked Nutrient

Water is crucial. It helps regulate body temperature, transport nutrients, and remove waste. Women should aim for about 2.7 liters of fluids per day, which can come from both drinks and water-rich foods (like fruits and vegetables). If you exercise or live in a hot climate, you may need more.

2.6 Balance and Moderation

When people say "balanced diet," it typically means a combination of carbohydrates, proteins, and fats, along with vitamins and minerals in proper amounts. It also means not eating too much of one food group at the expense of others. No single food can provide all the nutrients you need. That is why variety is key.

2.7 Reading Nutrition Labels

Learning to read **Nutrition Facts** labels can be a big help. In many countries, food packages list the serving size, total calories, and a breakdown of nutrients (fat, sodium, carbohydrates, sugars, protein, vitamins, and minerals). Here are some tips:

1. **Check Serving Size**: If you eat double the serving size, you get double the calories and nutrients.
2. **Look for Added Sugars**: Foods high in added sugars can spike blood sugar and add empty calories.
3. **Mind the Sodium**: Too much sodium can affect blood pressure. Look for lower-sodium options or rinse canned foods to reduce salt.
4. **Ingredients List**: Ingredients are listed in order of weight. If sugar or salt is near the top, the food might not be the healthiest choice.

2.8 The Role of Nutrient Density

Nutrient density means how many vitamins, minerals, and other beneficial substances a food provides compared to its calorie content. Foods like vegetables, fruits, whole grains, lean proteins, and low-fat dairy are usually high in nutrient density. Foods like sugary drinks, candy, and chips are low in nutrient density—they have many calories but few beneficial nutrients.

2.9 Energy Balance: Input vs. Output

Energy balance refers to matching the calories you eat (input) with the calories you burn (output). If you eat the same amount of calories that you burn, you will likely maintain your weight. If you eat fewer calories, you will usually lose weight, and if you eat more, you may gain weight. But keep in mind that weight is not the only measure of health. Body composition (ratio of muscle to fat) is also important.

2.10 Special Considerations for Women

1. **Iron Intake**: Women of childbearing age need more iron to replace what is lost during menstruation.
2. **Calcium and Vitamin D**: Important for bone health, especially since women are at higher risk for osteoporosis.
3. **Folic Acid (Folate)**: Crucial for women who might become pregnant, as it helps prevent certain birth defects.
4. **Healthy Fats**: Omega-3 fatty acids (found in fish, chia seeds, flaxseeds) support heart health and may help reduce inflammation.

2.11 Common Mistakes in Understanding Nutrition

- **Relying on a Single Food**: No single food (not even kale or quinoa) can meet all your needs. Variety is essential.
- **Skipping Meals**: Some people think eating less often is the key to weight loss. However, skipping meals can lead to overeating later.
- **Too Much of a Good Thing**: Even healthy foods can be over-consumed. Portion control still matters.
- **Falling for Fad Diets**: Trendy diets that cut out entire food groups might lead to short-term results, but often lack balanced nutrition.

2.12 Putting It into Practice

Let's look at a simple day's meal plan that follows basic nutrition principles:

- **Breakfast**: Oatmeal topped with berries and a tablespoon of peanut butter.
    - Provides complex carbs, some protein, and fiber.
- **Snack**: A piece of fruit (like an apple) or a small handful of almonds.
    - Gives extra vitamins, minerals, and healthy fats.
- **Lunch**: A salad with mixed greens, grilled chicken, avocado, tomatoes, and a light dressing.
    - Offers protein, healthy fats, fiber, and various vitamins.
- **Snack**: Low-fat yogurt or a small portion of cottage cheese with sliced bananas.
    - Another source of protein and calcium.
- **Dinner**: Salmon, brown rice, and steamed broccoli.
    - High-quality protein, complex carbs, healthy fats, and fiber.
- **Optional Dessert**: A small square of dark chocolate.
    - Offers antioxidants and satisfies sweet cravings in moderation.

2.13 Why "Dicts" Can Be Confusing

The term "diet" is sometimes misunderstood. It can mean:

1. **What you eat every day**—your general eating pattern.
2. **A restrictive plan** designed to lose weight quickly.

This book focuses on the first meaning—your overall eating pattern. We discourage fad diets that drastically cut calories or eliminate entire food groups (unless you have a medical reason). Extreme approaches often fail because they are not sustainable. Instead, aim for a balanced, long-term eating pattern that you can stick to.

2.14 The Importance of Listening to Your Body

Sometimes, we rely too much on external rules (like meal times, portion sizes on a package, or a random calorie target). While guidelines are helpful, it's also important to listen to hunger and fullness cues. Over time, practicing mindful eating can help you recognize when you are hungry, when you are satisfied, and when you are eating out of boredom or stress.

2.15 Tracking Your Progress

If you are trying to change your eating habits, you might benefit from a food diary or an app. Writing down what you eat can show patterns, such as whether you tend to overeat at night or if you skip breakfast. It can also help you be more mindful of food choices. However, do not let tracking become an obsession. The purpose is to understand patterns, not to judge yourself harshly.

2.16 Meal Timing

Some people find it helpful to eat small, frequent meals. Others do well with three main meals a day. There is no single right answer. What matters most is the total amount and balance of nutrients you take in over the course of a day or week. Experiment to see what makes you feel energized and satisfied.

2.17 Hydration and Drink Choices

Your body needs plenty of fluids. Water is usually the best choice, but there are other options:

- **Herbal Teas**: Can provide flavor and hydration without added calories or caffeine (depending on the blend).

- **Milk or Milk Alternatives**: Offer calcium and other nutrients. Watch out for added sugars in flavored varieties.
- **Fruit Juices**: Can be part of a healthy diet in small amounts, but they usually contain a lot of sugar. Choose 100% fruit juice and keep an eye on portion sizes.

Try to limit sugary drinks like soda or sweetened coffees, as they can lead to weight gain and spikes in blood sugar.

2.18 Addressing Dietary Restrictions

Many women have different dietary needs or restrictions:

- **Vegetarian or Vegan**: Focus on plant-based proteins (beans, lentils, tofu, tempeh), and make sure to get enough iron, calcium, and vitamin B12.
- **Gluten-Free**: Necessary for those with celiac disease or gluten intolerance. Many gluten-free products exist, but still pay attention to overall nutrient balance.
- **Lactose Intolerance**: Choose lactose-free dairy or alternatives like almond, soy, or oat milk. Check for calcium and vitamin D fortification.

2.19 Creating a Positive Relationship with Food

It is easy to develop a negative view of food when you are surrounded by diet advertisements. But remember, food is not the enemy. It is your source of nourishment. Try to focus on what you can add to your diet (more fruits, more veggies) instead of what you must remove. This positive mindset can help reduce feelings of deprivation.

CHAPTER 3: NUTRIENTS FOR WOMEN'S HEALTH

3.1 Why Certain Nutrients Are Extra Important for Women

Women's bodies have unique needs. For example, the menstrual cycle, pregnancy, breastfeeding, and menopause are all special phases. During these times, certain nutrients might be more critical. In addition, women often face a higher risk of conditions like iron deficiency and osteoporosis. Because of these issues, it is helpful to understand which nutrients can support overall health and help prevent or manage common concerns.

While Chapter 2 introduced the idea of macronutrients (carbohydrates, proteins, and fats) and micronutrients (vitamins and minerals), this chapter will focus on certain standout nutrients for women. We will discuss how they work in the body and why they matter. We will also look at helpful foods and easy ways to include these nutrients in your daily life.

3.2 Fiber and Its Benefits

Fiber is a type of carbohydrate that the body does not fully break down. Instead of turning into usable energy like other carbs, most fiber passes through the digestive system. Even though it is not "digested," fiber provides many benefits:

1. **Supports Healthy Digestion**: Fiber helps move food through the digestive tract. It can reduce constipation and support regular bowel movements.
2. **Helps Maintain a Healthy Weight**: Foods high in fiber tend to be more filling. This can help control hunger and prevent overeating.

3. **Regulates Blood Sugar**: Fiber slows down how quickly your body absorbs sugar from foods, helping keep blood sugar levels stable.
4. **Lowers Cholesterol**: Some types of fiber (soluble fiber) can help reduce LDL ("bad") cholesterol levels, which supports heart health.

3.2.1 Where to Find Fiber

- **Whole Grains**: Oats, whole wheat bread, brown rice, barley
- **Legumes**: Beans, lentils, chickpeas
- **Fruits**: Apples, berries, pears
- **Vegetables**: Broccoli, carrots, peas
- **Nuts and Seeds**: Almonds, chia seeds, flaxseeds

3.2.2 Tips for Getting Enough Fiber

- Start your day with a high-fiber breakfast, like oatmeal or whole-grain cereal.
- Choose whole-grain bread instead of white bread.
- Add beans or lentils to soups, salads, or main dishes.
- Snack on fruits and nuts instead of chips or sugary treats.

Fiber requirements vary, but many guidelines suggest that adult women should aim for around 25 grams of fiber per day, though some experts recommend even more. Because fiber also helps with satiety (fullness), it can be a helpful tool for weight management. However, increase fiber slowly if you are not used to it, and remember to drink plenty of water to help your body handle the extra bulk.

3.3 Antioxidants and Their Role in Women's Health

Antioxidants are molecules that help fight damage caused by free radicals. Free radicals are unstable molecules that can harm cells in our bodies. This damage is linked to aging, inflammation, and various diseases. Women may benefit from antioxidants because these nutrients can help reduce inflammation and protect cells.

3.3.1 Common Antioxidants

1. **Vitamin C**: Found in citrus fruits, strawberries, bell peppers, and broccoli.
2. **Vitamin E**: Found in nuts, seeds, and vegetable oils.
3. **Beta-Carotene**: Found in orange-colored fruits and vegetables like carrots, sweet potatoes, and cantaloupe.
4. **Selenium**: A mineral found in Brazil nuts, sunflower seeds, and certain types of fish.
5. **Polyphenols**: Found in tea (green, black), berries, dark chocolate, and olives.

3.3.2 Benefits of Antioxidants for Women

- **Skin Health**: Many women are concerned about skin aging. Antioxidants can support skin by helping reduce cell damage from the sun and the environment.
- **Cell Repair**: By protecting cells from free-radical damage, antioxidants may aid in overall repair.
- **Disease Prevention**: Research suggests that a diet high in antioxidant-rich foods may help lower the risk of chronic diseases, such as heart disease and certain cancers.

3.4 Phytonutrients: The Special Compounds in Plants

Beyond vitamins and minerals, plants contain thousands of special compounds known as **phytonutrients**. These are not considered essential in the same way vitamins or minerals are, but they can provide health benefits. Phytonutrients often give fruits and vegetables their vibrant colors. Examples include:

- **Lycopene** (in tomatoes and watermelon)
- **Lutein** (in leafy greens)
- **Anthocyanins** (in berries and purple cabbage)

These compounds may help with different aspects of health, such as eye health, heart function, and even cognitive function. Eating a wide range of colorful fruits and vegetables is one of the best ways to get these beneficial phytonutrients.

3.5 Omega-3 Fatty Acids: Heart, Hormone, and Brain Benefits

Omega-3 fatty acids are a type of polyunsaturated fat that is often called a "good fat." They are especially important for women because they help support heart health, reduce inflammation, and may even help balance hormones. Some studies suggest that omega-3s can be beneficial during pregnancy for the baby's brain development, and they might help lessen menstrual discomfort for some women.

3.5.1 Where to Find Omega-3s

- **Fatty Fish**: Salmon, mackerel, sardines, trout
- **Chia Seeds and Flaxseeds**: Great sources of plant-based omega-3 (alpha-linolenic acid or ALA)
- **Walnuts**: Another plant source of ALA
- **Omega-3 Enriched Eggs**: Some eggs come from hens fed a diet high in omega-3s

Since many women do not eat enough fish, looking for ways to add more omega-3s to your diet can be beneficial. You can sprinkle ground flaxseeds or chia seeds on your oatmeal or salad. If fish is part of your diet, try aiming for two servings of fatty fish each week to meet your needs.

3.6 Probiotics and Gut Health

Probiotics are live bacteria and yeasts that are good for your digestive system. They are often called "good" or "friendly" bacteria because they can help keep your gut healthy. Women in particular can benefit from probiotics to support healthy digestion and potentially help with certain urinary or vaginal health concerns.

3.6.1 Sources of Probiotics

- **Yogurt with Live Cultures**
- **Kefir** (a fermented milk drink)
- **Sauerkraut** and Kimchi (fermented vegetables)
- **Kombucha** (fermented tea)
- **Tempeh** and Miso (fermented soy products)

A healthy gut microbiome—where these "good" bacteria live—may help in digestion and absorption of nutrients, support immune function, and possibly even influence mood. Although more research is ongoing, many doctors and nutrition experts suggest that including probiotic-rich foods can be a good step toward better overall health.

3.7 Iron: Preventing Deficiency

Iron is critical for making hemoglobin, a protein in red blood cells that carries oxygen throughout the body. Women need more iron than men, especially during the reproductive years, because of monthly blood loss through menstruation. Too little iron can lead to anemia, a condition that causes fatigue, weakness, and difficulty concentrating.

3.7.1 Best Sources of Iron

- **Heme Iron** (easiest for the body to absorb): Found in red meat, poultry, and fish.
- **Non-Heme Iron**: Found in beans, lentils, spinach, fortified cereals, and nuts.

To improve iron absorption, pair non-heme iron foods with vitamin C-rich foods (like orange juice or tomatoes). If you are a vegetarian or vegan, be extra mindful to include enough iron-rich foods every day and consider cooking in cast iron pans. Some women may need supplements, but it's best to check with a healthcare provider before adding an iron supplement.

3.8 Calcium for Strong Bones

Calcium is a key nutrient for building and maintaining strong bones. It also plays a role in muscle function and nerve signaling. Women are at higher risk for osteoporosis, especially after menopause, because lower estrogen levels can accelerate bone loss.

3.8.1 Best Sources of Calcium

- **Dairy Products**: Milk, cheese, yogurt
- **Fortified Plant Milks**: Almond, soy, oat milks (check labels for calcium content)
- **Leafy Green Vegetables**: Kale, collard greens, bok choy
- **Fortified Foods**: Certain cereals or orange juices may have added calcium

A good calcium intake, combined with weight-bearing exercise (like walking, jogging, or strength training), can help keep bones strong. Vitamin D also works closely with calcium for bone health, as it helps the body absorb calcium.

3.9 Vitamin D Synergy

Vitamin D is sometimes called the "sunshine vitamin" because our skin produces it when exposed to sunlight. However, many people—especially those who live in areas with long winters or who spend a lot of time indoors—may not get enough sun exposure to meet their needs. Vitamin D supports bone health, immune function, and may even have a role in mood regulation.

3.9.1 Sources of Vitamin D

- **Sun Exposure**: About 10-15 minutes of midday sun (without sunscreen) can help, but this varies by skin type, location, and time of year.
- **Fatty Fish**: Salmon, mackerel, sardines
- **Fortified Dairy or Plant Milks**
- **Egg Yolks**

Because many women do not get enough vitamin D from food or sunlight alone, some turn to supplements. If you think you might be low in vitamin D, you can get a blood test to check your level. The right amount of vitamin D helps with calcium absorption, which is vital for healthy bones.

3.10 Magnesium: The "Helper" Mineral

Magnesium is involved in hundreds of chemical reactions in the body. It helps with muscle relaxation, nerve function, and energy production. Some women find that adequate magnesium intake can help ease muscle cramps or discomfort during PMS (premenstrual syndrome).

3.10.1 Magnesium-Rich Foods

- **Dark Leafy Greens**: Spinach, Swiss chard
- **Nuts and Seeds**: Almonds, pumpkin seeds, sunflower seeds
- **Whole Grains**: Brown rice, whole wheat bread
- **Beans and Legumes**

A varied diet with plenty of whole foods often meets magnesium needs. However, certain health conditions or medications can affect magnesium absorption or excretion, so it's good to pay attention to signs of low magnesium, such as muscle cramps or fatigue. Always check with a healthcare professional for personalized advice.

3.11 Protein Quality for Women

We already talked about protein in Chapter 2, but let's focus on what "quality" means. Women who are pregnant, breastfeeding, or trying to build muscle might need more protein. Protein sources vary in their amino acid profiles:

- **Lean Meat, Poultry, and Fish**: Complete proteins with all essential amino acids.
- **Eggs**: Also a complete protein. One egg provides about 6 grams of high-quality protein.
- **Dairy**: Milk, cheese, and yogurt can be good sources if you eat dairy.
- **Plant-Based Protein**: Beans, lentils, tofu, tempeh, nuts, and seeds.

Combining plant-based foods (like rice and beans) can give you a complete amino acid profile. This is helpful for vegetarians or vegans who want to ensure they get all essential amino acids.

3.12 Hydration: A Nutrient Often Forgotten

We often think of nutrients as vitamins, minerals, or fiber, but **water** is also crucial. Dehydration can cause headaches, fatigue, and trouble concentrating. Women who are active or live in warm climates may need more fluids. While Chapter 2 briefly introduced water, here we want to remind you that staying properly hydrated helps with:

- **Temperature Regulation**
- **Nutrient Transport**
- **Healthy Skin**
- **Digestion**

Try to keep a reusable water bottle handy. If plain water seems boring, you can add slices of lemon, cucumber, or berries to add flavor without extra sugar.

3.13 Putting It All Together: Creating Balanced Meals

Now that we have looked at several special nutrients for women's health, let's consider how to combine them into daily eating. A balanced meal might look like this:

- **Protein** (chicken, fish, tofu, or beans)
- **High-Fiber Carbohydrates** (whole grains, sweet potatoes, or legumes)
- **Colorful Veggies** (to get antioxidants and phytonutrients)
- **Healthy Fats** (avocado, nuts, seeds, or olive oil)
- **Calcium Source** (milk, fortified plant milk, or a leafy green side dish)

For example, a simple dinner could be grilled salmon (protein + omega-3s) with brown rice (whole grain) and steamed broccoli (antioxidants + fiber). You might add a small side salad with spinach (iron) and a sprinkle of nuts (healthy fats + magnesium). This combination covers many nutrients beneficial for women's health.

3.14 Small Changes for Big Benefits

Sometimes the idea of "eating healthy" can feel overwhelming. However, making small shifts in your daily routine can have a lasting impact:

- **Add a serving of vegetables** to at least two meals per day.
- **Swap refined grains** for whole grains (e.g., white rice to brown rice).
- **Try a new fruit** each week to get different antioxidants.
- **Include legumes** (beans, lentils) a few times a week.
- **Limit processed snacks** that offer little nutritional value.

You do not have to change everything at once. Pick one or two habits you want to focus on, then build from there.

3.15 Nutrient Timing and Women's Hormonal Cycles

Women's hormonal cycles can affect appetite, cravings, and energy levels. Some women notice they crave more carbohydrates or sugary foods just before their period. Others feel more tired and might need extra iron or magnesium. Paying attention to your body and planning ahead can help:

- **Pre-Menstrual**: Increase magnesium-rich foods (nuts, seeds, leafy greens) and keep healthy snacks on hand.
- **During Menstruation**: Ensure sufficient iron from sources like lean meats, beans, or fortified cereals.
- **Throughout the Month**: Focus on balance, variety, and staying hydrated.

3.16 Common Pitfalls and How to Avoid Them

1. **Relying Too Much on Supplements**: While vitamins and minerals in pill form can be helpful, they are not a substitute for whole foods. Real foods contain fiber, antioxidants, and phytonutrients that supplements do not fully replicate.
2. **Skipping Meals**: Skipping meals might lead to overeating later or choosing less nutritious foods on the go.
3. **Overly Restricting Foods**: Cutting out entire groups (like carbs or fats) can lead to imbalances in your diet.
4. **Ignoring Liquid Calories**: Sugary drinks can add a lot of calories without the nutritional benefits.
5. **Underestimating Calcium and Vitamin D Needs**: Especially important for bone health, yet often overlooked.

3.17 Signs You Might Need More Specific Nutrients

- **Iron**: Constant fatigue, pale skin, brittle nails might suggest anemia.
- **Calcium**: Weak nails, muscle cramps, or a history of fractures might be signs you need more calcium (or vitamin D).
- **Magnesium**: Muscle cramps, trouble sleeping, or stress overload could point to low magnesium.
- **Omega-3s**: Very dry skin, excessive inflammation, or certain mood issues might improve with more omega-3s.

If you suspect a nutrient deficiency, talk to a healthcare provider. A blood test can confirm if you really are deficient in iron, vitamin D, or something else. Then you can work on a plan to correct it through diet and possible supplements.

CHAPTER 4: VITAMINS, MINERALS, AND OTHER MICRONUTRIENTS

4.1 Introduction to Micronutrients

In Chapter 3, we took a closer look at key nutrients that play a large role in women's health. In this chapter, we will explore **vitamins**, **minerals**, and other **micronutrients** more systematically. Micronutrients do not provide calories the way carbohydrates, proteins, or fats do, but they are essential for many bodily functions. They help with energy production, immune support, hormone regulation, and more.

Women often have unique needs for certain vitamins and minerals, such as iron, calcium, and folate. We'll break down the main vitamins (A, B, C, D, E, K) and important minerals (like calcium, iron, magnesium, zinc) and also discuss other helpful substances like choline and iodine. This chapter will help you understand why each micronutrient matters, how much you might need, and how to find it in everyday foods.

4.2 The Fat-Soluble Vitamins (A, D, E, K)

Fat-soluble vitamins dissolve in fat and are stored in the body's fatty tissues and liver. Because they can be stored, you do not have to consume them every single day, but it's still good to keep up a regular intake.

4.2.1 Vitamin A

- **Role**: Supports eye health, immune function, and cell growth.

- **Sources**: Beta-carotene in carrots, sweet potatoes, spinach, and cantaloupe converts to vitamin A in the body. Preformed vitamin A is found in eggs, liver, and fortified dairy products.
- **Women's Health Angle**: Adequate vitamin A is crucial during pregnancy for fetal development, but too much (especially from supplements) can cause problems.

4.2.2 Vitamin D

- **Role**: Aids in calcium absorption, important for bones and immune function.
- **Sources**: Sunlight exposure helps your body produce vitamin D. It's also found in fatty fish (salmon, sardines), fortified milk, and some mushrooms.
- **Women's Health Angle**: Women need to watch their vitamin D levels for strong bones, especially as they age.

4.2.3 Vitamin E

- **Role**: Acts as an antioxidant, supports cell function, and helps the immune system.
- **Sources**: Nuts, seeds (especially sunflower seeds, almonds), vegetable oils, and spinach.
- **Women's Health Angle**: Some studies suggest vitamin E might help relieve menstrual discomfort or support skin health, but more research is needed.

4.2.4 Vitamin K

- **Role**: Helps with blood clotting and bone health.
- **Sources**: Leafy green vegetables (kale, spinach, collard greens), broccoli, and Brussels sprouts.
- **Women's Health Angle**: Works with vitamin D and calcium to maintain strong bones, which is important to prevent osteoporosis.

4.3 The Water-Soluble Vitamins (B Complex & Vitamin C)

Water-soluble vitamins dissolve in water and are not stored in large amounts in the body. You need a regular supply of these vitamins to stay healthy.

4.3.1 B Vitamins Overview

- **Types**: B1 (thiamin), B2 (riboflavin), B3 (niacin), B5 (pantothenic acid), B6 (pyridoxine), B7 (biotin), B9 (folate or folic acid), B12 (cobalamin).
- **Role**: Each B vitamin has its own function, but together they help convert food into energy, support nerve function, and help form red blood cells.

4.3.1.1 Folate (Vitamin B9)

- **Why It Matters**: Essential for cell growth and making DNA. This is crucial for pregnant women to prevent certain birth defects (like spina bifida).
- **Sources**: Leafy greens, legumes, fortified cereals, and citrus fruits.
- **Women's Health Angle**: All women of childbearing age are often encouraged to consume enough folate or take a folic acid supplement if they might become pregnant.

4.3.1.2 Vitamin B12 (Cobalamin)

- **Why It Matters**: Helps keep nerves and blood cells healthy, aids in DNA production.
- **Sources**: Primarily found in animal products like meat, fish, poultry, eggs, and dairy. Fortified cereals and nutritional yeast can provide B12 for vegetarians or vegans.
- **Women's Health Angle**: Vegetarians, vegans, and older women may be at higher risk for B12 deficiency, which can cause tiredness and nerve problems.

4.3.2 Vitamin C

- **Role**: Supports immune function, acts as an antioxidant, helps with collagen production (important for skin and connective tissues).
- **Sources**: Citrus fruits (oranges, grapefruit), berries (strawberries, raspberries), bell peppers, and broccoli.
- **Women's Health Angle**: Vitamin C helps with iron absorption, a key point for women who need more iron. It also supports skin health and wound healing, which can be especially helpful for women after childbirth or surgeries.

4.4 Important Minerals for Women

4.4.1 Calcium

Chapter 3 covered calcium for bone health. Just to recap:

- **Role**: Builds bones and teeth, helps with muscle contraction, and supports nerve function.
- **Sources**: Dairy, fortified plant milks, leafy greens.
- **Women's Health Angle**: Essential to prevent osteoporosis, especially after menopause when bone loss speeds up.

4.4.2 Iron

As mentioned in Chapter 3, iron is vital for women. Quick summary:

- **Role**: Carries oxygen in the blood, needed for energy.
- **Sources**: Red meat, poultry, fish, beans, spinach, fortified cereals.
- **Women's Health Angle**: Menstruation increases the risk of iron deficiency.

4.4.3 Magnesium

Also noted in Chapter 3, magnesium supports muscle and nerve function, among other things. Quick points:

- **Role**: Helps with hundreds of enzymatic reactions in the body, including energy production.
- **Sources**: Leafy greens, nuts, seeds, whole grains, legumes.
- **Women's Health Angle**: May help reduce cramps and PMS symptoms.

4.4.4 Zinc

- **Role**: Supports immune function, wound healing, and DNA synthesis. Also helps with taste and smell.
- **Sources**: Red meat, poultry, beans, nuts, whole grains, fortified cereals.
- **Women's Health Angle**: Adequate zinc supports a healthy immune system and might help with skin health. During pregnancy, zinc is crucial for fetal development.

4.4.5 Iodine

- **Role**: Needed to make thyroid hormones, which control metabolism and growth.
- **Sources**: Iodized salt, seafood, dairy, and certain breads.
- **Women's Health Angle**: Very important during pregnancy for the baby's brain development. Low iodine can lead to thyroid problems, which may affect energy and weight.

4.5 Other Helpful Micronutrients and Substances

4.5.1 Choline

- **Role**: Supports liver function, brain development, and nerve function.
- **Sources**: Eggs (specifically egg yolks), meat, fish, dairy, and certain beans.

- **Women's Health Angle**: Important during pregnancy for fetal brain development. Many women do not get enough choline, so including choline-rich foods or a prenatal vitamin with choline can be helpful if you are pregnant.

4.5.2 Selenium

- **Role**: Works as an antioxidant and supports thyroid function.
- **Sources**: Brazil nuts are especially high in selenium, along with seafood and some meats.
- **Women's Health Angle**: Supports immune health and proper thyroid function, which is crucial for women because thyroid issues are more common in women than in men.

4.5.3 Chromium

- **Role**: Helps with insulin function and regulating blood sugar levels.
- **Sources**: Whole grains, broccoli, and lean meats.
- **Women's Health Angle**: Some research suggests that chromium may support normal blood sugar balance, which could be important for women dealing with conditions like polycystic ovary syndrome (PCOS).

4.6 Meeting Your Micronutrient Needs Through Food

The best way to ensure you get enough vitamins and minerals is by eating a variety of nutrient-dense foods:

1. **Colorful Plates**: Fruits and vegetables of different colors provide different vitamins and antioxidants.
2. **Whole Grains**: Brown rice, oats, and whole wheat contain more B vitamins and minerals than refined grains.
3. **Lean Proteins**: Fish, poultry, beans, lentils, eggs, and lean meats help you get B vitamins, iron, zinc, and more.
4. **Low-Fat Dairy or Fortified Alternatives**: Gives you calcium, vitamin D, and often vitamin B12.

5. **Nuts and Seeds**: Provide healthy fats, magnesium, vitamin E, and other minerals.

4.7 When Might Supplements Be Necessary?

Although whole foods should be your main source of nutrients, some women may need supplements in certain cases:

- **Pregnancy**: Folic acid, iron, choline, and prenatal vitamins are common.
- **Vegan or Vegetarian Diets**: Vitamin B12, iron, or vitamin D supplements might be required if you are not getting enough from food.
- **Food Allergies**: If you avoid certain foods (like dairy), you might need calcium or vitamin D supplements.
- **Medical Conditions**: Certain digestive disorders, thyroid issues, or other health problems might affect how your body absorbs nutrients.

Always talk to a healthcare provider or a registered dietitian before starting a supplement. Taking too much of certain vitamins or minerals can cause harm. For example, fat-soluble vitamins (A, D, E, and K) can build up in your body if taken in excess.

4.8 Recognizing Deficiencies and Imbalances

Micronutrient deficiencies can be sneaky. Some people might feel tired all the time and not realize they are low in iron or B12. Others might experience muscle cramps and not suspect low magnesium. If you have symptoms that persist—like extreme fatigue, hair loss, frequent colds, or brittle nails—it might be worth talking to a healthcare provider. Blood tests can often reveal deficiencies, and then you can work on a plan to fix them.

4.9 The Dangers of Over-Supplementation

While many people worry about deficiencies, it is also possible to get too much of a good thing. Taking high doses of vitamins and minerals (especially from supplements) can lead to imbalances or toxicity. For example:

- **Vitamin A Toxicity**: Can cause headaches, dizziness, and even serious liver problems in extreme cases.
- **Iron Overload**: Can damage organs if levels get too high.
- **Calcium Excess**: May lead to kidney stones or interfere with how other minerals are absorbed.

It's best to prioritize real foods and only use supplements if your diet or condition truly requires it.

4.10 Micronutrients Across Different Life Stages

Women's needs for vitamins and minerals change over time:

1. **Teens and Young Adults**: Need extra calcium and vitamin D for bone development. Iron is also important during menstruation.
2. **Pregnancy**: Folate, iron, calcium, and choline are critical.
3. **Breastfeeding**: Requires a bit more of most nutrients to support milk production.
4. **Menopause and Beyond**: Calcium, vitamin D, magnesium, and vitamin B12 become more crucial, as hormone changes can affect bone density and nutrient absorption.

4.11 Micronutrients and Skin, Hair, and Nails

Many women care about the health of their skin, hair, and nails. Micronutrients often play a big role here:

- **Vitamin C**: Supports collagen, which is important for skin elasticity.
- **Biotin (Vitamin B7)**: Linked to healthy hair and nails.
- **Zinc**: Helps with wound healing and may reduce acne.
- **Omega-3 Fatty Acids**: Not a vitamin or mineral but can support skin moisture and reduce dryness.

If you are experiencing skin or hair problems, checking your nutrient intake might be helpful, along with looking at other factors like stress, hormones, and overall diet.

4.12 Stress and Micronutrient Needs

Stress can impact how your body uses nutrients. When you are stressed, you might burn through certain vitamins and minerals faster, especially the B vitamins and magnesium. Stress hormones can also affect appetite and digestion, either reducing your desire to eat or leading you to overeat less nutritious foods. During stressful times, making sure you have balanced meals and possibly including stress-busting nutrients (like magnesium) can be beneficial.

4.13 Interactions Between Micronutrients

Vitamins and minerals often work together or affect how the body uses them:

- **Vitamin C and Iron**: Vitamin C boosts iron absorption, especially non-heme iron from plant sources.
- **Calcium and Vitamin D**: Vitamin D helps your body absorb calcium.
- **Iron and Calcium**: Taking high doses of both at the same time can reduce absorption of each. That's why some doctors recommend spacing them out during the day.

Understanding these interactions can help you plan meals or time supplements to get the best effect.

4.14 Simple Ways to Increase Micronutrient Intake

1. **Add More Veggies to Your Plate**: Mix chopped peppers, onions, or spinach into your eggs. Add grated carrots or zucchini into pasta sauce.
2. **Choose Whole Grains**: Swap white bread for whole wheat or refine your usual recipes with whole-grain alternatives.
3. **Snack on Fruit**: Instead of chips or cookies, choose an apple, pear, or berries for antioxidants and vitamins.
4. **Fortified Foods**: Choose cereals or plant milks fortified with B12, vitamin D, or calcium if your diet is lacking in these areas.
5. **Include a Salad**: A big mixed salad with colorful vegetables, beans, seeds, and a protein source can cover many micronutrients in one meal.

4.15 Meal Examples Rich in Micronutrients

- **Breakfast**: Whole grain toast with peanut butter (vitamin E, healthy fats), a bowl of mixed berries (vitamin C, antioxidants), and a glass of fortified orange juice (calcium, vitamin D).
- **Lunch**: Spinach salad with grilled chicken (iron, protein), sliced strawberries (vitamin C), walnuts (omega-3s, magnesium), and a light vinaigrette.
- **Dinner**: Baked salmon (vitamin D, omega-3s), sweet potato (beta-carotene, fiber), and steamed broccoli (vitamin C, potassium).
- **Snack**: Yogurt with live cultures (probiotics, calcium) and a drizzle of honey or fresh fruit.

4.16 Addressing Special Diets

1. **Vegetarian/Vegan**: Pay close attention to B12, iron, zinc, and calcium. Fortified foods and a variety of plant-based proteins can help.

2. **Gluten-Free**: Choose naturally gluten-free whole grains like quinoa, brown rice, or buckwheat to still get B vitamins and minerals.
3. **Dairy-Free**: Make sure you have calcium and vitamin D from fortified plant milks, leafy greens, and possibly supplements if recommended by a doctor.

4.17 Micronutrient Myths

1. **"All Supplements Are Safe."** Not necessarily. Some can interact with medications or cause toxicity if overused.
2. **"You Only Need Supplements When You're Older."** Younger women might also need certain supplements if their diet is lacking.
3. **"Natural Is Always Better."** Natural or synthetic, your body often sees the vitamin the same way. But focusing on real, whole foods is still the best first choice.
4. **"Vitamin C Cures the Common Cold."** It can support immune health, but it is not a guaranteed cure.

4.18 Checking Labels and Serving Sizes

If you choose to use supplements:

- Look for brands that are tested by third parties (like USP or NSF) to ensure quality.
- Check the serving size. Sometimes a supplement will say "2 capsules per serving," which changes how much you actually take.
- Be mindful of the daily recommended values. Don't automatically go for mega-doses.

4.19 The Bigger Picture: Balancing Food and Lifestyle

Micronutrients do not work in isolation. Your body needs an overall balanced diet, plus a healthy lifestyle that includes:

- **Regular Physical Activity**: Helps maintain a healthy weight and can improve mood, which might reduce stress eating.
- **Adequate Sleep**: Sleep is when your body repairs and regenerates cells. Not getting enough rest can affect how your body uses nutrients.
- **Stress Management**: Chronic stress can deplete certain nutrients. Relaxation techniques (like deep breathing, meditation, or yoga) might help your nutrient balance.

4.20 Key Takeaways from Chapter 4

1. **Micronutrients** are vital for health even though they do not provide calories.
2. **Fat-Soluble Vitamins (A, D, E, K)** can be stored in the body, so be careful not to over-supplement.
3. **Water-Soluble Vitamins (B Complex, C)** need regular replenishment. B9 (folate) is especially crucial for women of childbearing age.
4. **Important Minerals** like calcium, iron, magnesium, and zinc have special roles in women's health.
5. **Other Substances** like choline and selenium also contribute to overall well-being.
6. **Food First**: Aim to meet needs through a varied diet of whole foods, and supplement only if needed.
7. **Life Stages** influence micronutrient needs—pregnancy, lactation, and menopause require different amounts.
8. **Avoid Overdoing It**: Excess intake of certain vitamins or minerals can be harmful.
9. **Lifestyle Factors**—such as sleep, stress, and exercise—affect how your body uses these nutrients.

By learning how vitamins and minerals work together, you can make smart food choices that support your body's natural processes. From boosting your immune system and energy levels to supporting strong bones and healthy skin, micronutrients are truly the unsung heroes of a balanced diet.

CHAPTER 5: HORMONES AND HOW THEY AFFECT NUTRITION

5.1 Basic Hormone Facts

Hormones are chemical messengers in the body. They are made by different glands and travel through the bloodstream to tell cells or organs what to do. Women have a unique hormonal system that shifts during the menstrual cycle, pregnancy, and menopause. Because hormones can influence how we feel, how we eat, and how we process nutrients, understanding them is important for overall health.

In earlier chapters, we talked about nutrients, vitamins, and minerals. Now, we turn to hormones. Hormones interact with the foods you eat. For example, what you eat can affect insulin levels in your body, or it may help keep estrogen and other hormones in balance. By seeing the whole picture—both nutrition and hormone function—women can better manage weight, mood swings, energy levels, and more.

5.2 Major Hormones in Women's Bodies

There are several key hormones that play big roles in a woman's health and nutrition. Here are the main ones we will focus on:

1. **Estrogen**
2. **Progesterone**
3. **Testosterone** (yes, women have it too, just in smaller amounts)
4. **Thyroid Hormones**
5. **Insulin**

6. **Cortisol**

Each one has a particular job, and they often work together or counterbalance each other.

5.2.1 Estrogen

Estrogen is often called the "primary female hormone." It supports female reproductive functions, helps regulate the menstrual cycle, and affects bone health. It also influences where fat is stored in the body (often around the hips and thighs for women).

- **Where It Comes From**: Mostly produced by the ovaries, but also in small amounts by the adrenal glands and fat tissue.
- **Nutritional Impact**: Fluctuating estrogen can change appetite and cravings. Low estrogen levels, especially after menopause, can speed up bone loss, increasing the need for calcium and vitamin D.

5.2.2 Progesterone

Progesterone works with estrogen to regulate the menstrual cycle. Levels typically rise in the second half of the cycle (the luteal phase) after ovulation.

- **Where It Comes From**: Produced by the corpus luteum in the ovary after ovulation and by the placenta during pregnancy.
- **Nutritional Impact**: Changes in progesterone may influence mood and water retention. Some women feel bloated or experience food cravings in the luteal phase.

5.2.3 Testosterone

Yes, women produce testosterone, though much less than men. Testosterone helps with libido (sex drive), bone strength, and building muscle mass.

- **Where It Comes From**: Made by the ovaries and adrenal glands.
- **Nutritional Impact**: Very low levels might result in reduced muscle mass or energy. Eating enough protein and certain nutrients (like zinc) can help maintain healthy levels.

5.2.4 Thyroid Hormones

The thyroid gland in your neck makes hormones (mainly T3 and T4) that control how fast your body uses energy—your metabolism.

- **Where They Come From**: The thyroid gland, regulated by the pituitary gland in the brain.
- **Nutritional Impact**: If thyroid hormone levels are low (hypothyroidism), you might feel tired and gain weight more easily. If they are high (hyperthyroidism), you might feel anxious or lose weight quickly. Iodine and selenium are among the nutrients important for thyroid function.

5.2.5 Insulin

Insulin helps your cells take in glucose (sugar) from your bloodstream, providing energy. It's essential for controlling blood sugar levels.

- **Where It Comes From**: The pancreas.
- **Nutritional Impact**: Eating too many simple carbohydrates at once can spike blood sugar and insulin. Over time, this can lead to insulin resistance, a risk factor for conditions like type 2 diabetes and certain hormonal imbalances (such as polycystic ovary syndrome, or PCOS).

5.2.6 Cortisol

Cortisol is known as the "stress hormone." It's released by the adrenal glands when you're under physical or emotional stress.

- **Where It Comes From**: The adrenal glands (just above the kidneys).
- **Nutritional Impact**: Chronic stress can raise cortisol levels, which might increase cravings for high-sugar or high-fat foods. Over time, high cortisol can affect weight, especially around the abdomen.

5.3 Hormonal Fluctuations During the Menstrual Cycle

A typical menstrual cycle is about 28 days, though it can range from 21 to 35 days. Hormone levels change throughout these phases:

1. **Menstrual Phase (Days 1–5)**: Estrogen and progesterone are low. You might feel more tired.
2. **Follicular Phase (Days 1–13)**: Estrogen begins to rise. This can often boost mood and energy.
3. **Ovulation (Day 14 in a 28-day cycle)**: Estrogen peaks, and luteinizing hormone (LH) triggers the release of an egg. Some women might feel more energetic or have a higher libido.
4. **Luteal Phase (Days 15–28)**: Progesterone increases, and estrogen drops slightly. Some women may experience cravings, bloating, or moodiness (PMS) before the next period begins.

Understanding these phases can help you adjust your eating patterns. For instance, during the luteal phase, you might want to focus on magnesium-rich foods (like nuts and leafy greens) to help manage cramps or cravings.

5.4 The Link Between Hormones and Appetite

Hormones like **ghrelin** (hunger hormone) and **leptin** (satiety hormone) also play roles in a woman's appetite. While these hormones aren't female-specific, they can be influenced by other hormonal changes. For example, in the days before your period, you might notice a stronger desire for carbohydrate-rich or sweet foods.

Some research suggests that the fluctuations of estrogen and progesterone can impact leptin, leading to more cravings.

Practical Tips:

- Keep healthy snacks around if you tend to crave sweets or salty foods before your period.
- Make sure you have balanced meals with protein, fiber, and healthy fats to promote longer-lasting fullness.
- Pay attention to emotional triggers. Stress can heighten hunger signals even if your body does not truly need more energy.

5.5 Hormones and Weight

Weight management can be complex for women because hormones often shift throughout life—puberty, pregnancy, postpartum, perimenopause, and menopause. Hormonal changes can affect appetite, metabolism, and even how your body stores fat.

- **Puberty**: Increased estrogen can lead to changes in body shape, with more fat stored in the hips and thighs.
- **Pregnancy**: Hormones help the body prepare to nurture a developing baby. Weight gain is natural and needed, but excessive weight gain can be harder to lose later.
- **Menopause**: As estrogen levels drop, fat storage might shift to the abdominal area, and metabolism can slow down.

In all these stages, a balanced diet, regular exercise, and stress management are vital. It's also helpful to understand that these changes are normal, and they may require you to adapt your eating patterns and activity levels over time.

5.6 Stress Hormones and Emotional Eating

When you face chronic stress, your body releases more cortisol. High cortisol levels can make you crave high-energy (often sugary or fatty) foods. This is because the body's stress response was originally meant to help you survive immediate dangers, so it encourages you to refuel in case you need energy to "fight or flee."

However, modern stress is often mental or emotional rather than physical. You might be stressed about work, finances, or relationships. The body doesn't always know the difference between facing a lion or facing a tough day at the office—it still pumps out cortisol.

Ways to Cope:

- Practice relaxation techniques (deep breathing, meditation, short walks).
- Keep healthy snack options available, like sliced fruit, nuts, or yogurt.
- Stay hydrated; thirst can sometimes feel like hunger.
- Talk to a counselor or friend if stress eating is a constant struggle.

5.7 Hormones and Sleep

Sleep is closely linked to hormones. Poor sleep affects ghrelin (making you hungrier) and leptin (making you feel less full). It can also elevate cortisol. When you're tired, you might reach for sugary foods or caffeine to boost energy. Over time, this creates a cycle of poor sleep and less healthy eating.

Try to maintain a sleep schedule: aim for 7 to 8 hours of rest per night. Good sleep habits (like reducing screen time before bed and limiting caffeine later in the day) can make a huge difference in hormone balance.

5.8 Balancing Hormones Through Nutrition

Food doesn't replace medical treatments, but certain choices can help support hormone balance:

1. **Focus on Whole Foods**: Fruits, vegetables, whole grains, lean proteins, and healthy fats.
2. **Limit Excess Sugar**: Too much sugar can spike insulin levels and may contribute to hormone imbalances over time.
3. **Include Protein** in each meal to stabilize blood sugar and assist with muscle maintenance.
4. **Healthy Fats** (like those from avocados, nuts, seeds, and fatty fish) support hormone production.
5. **Fiber-Rich Foods** help remove excess hormones from the body and keep digestion regular.

For example, if you have issues with estrogen dominance (too much estrogen relative to progesterone), a high-fiber diet with plenty of cruciferous vegetables (like broccoli, cauliflower, and Brussels sprouts) might help your body eliminate excess estrogen.

5.9 Foods That Support Hormonal Balance

Certain foods are often mentioned as helpful for hormone balance in women:

- **Flaxseeds**: Contain lignans, which may help modulate estrogen levels.
- **Cruciferous Vegetables**: Broccoli, kale, cabbage, cauliflower—these may support the liver's role in processing hormones.
- **Berries**: High in antioxidants, can help reduce inflammation.
- **Green Leafy Vegetables**: Provide magnesium, folate, and other nutrients beneficial for hormone health.

- **Fatty Fish**: Salmon, mackerel, and sardines offer omega-3 fatty acids, which can support hormone function and reduce inflammation.

Still, no single food is a magic bullet. It's the overall pattern that counts. Consistency in healthy eating—rather than one specific superfood—will yield better long-term benefits for hormone balance.

5.10 Lifestyle Habits for Healthy Hormones

Beyond eating well, these habits can help stabilize hormones:

1. **Regular Exercise**: Moderate physical activity (like brisk walking, light jogging, or strength training) can improve insulin sensitivity, support weight management, and reduce stress.
2. **Stress Management**: Chronic stress leads to chronically high cortisol, which can throw off other hormones. Mindful activities, hobbies, or just taking short breaks during the day can help.
3. **Adequate Sleep**: As mentioned, good sleep regulates appetite hormones and stress hormones.
4. **Limit Alcohol**: Excessive alcohol can disrupt hormone levels (like estrogen) and burden the liver, which is important for processing hormones.
5. **Avoid Smoking**: Smoking can affect estrogen levels, bone health, and overall hormone balance.

5.11 Special Considerations: PCOS and Thyroid Disorders

Some women have specific conditions like **polycystic ovary syndrome (PCOS)**, which involves insulin resistance and elevated androgens (male hormones). These women often experience irregular periods, acne, or weight gain. A balanced diet that moderates carb intake and focuses on whole foods can help manage insulin resistance.

Thyroid disorders (hypothyroidism or hyperthyroidism) can also affect weight, energy levels, and mood. If you suspect a thyroid issue—common signs include extreme tiredness, hair loss, sensitivity to cold (hypothyroidism) or feeling too warm, anxiety, and weight loss (hyperthyroidism)—talk with a healthcare professional. Your nutrition plan may need adjustments, such as enough iodine, selenium, and overall calorie intake based on your thyroid function.

5.12 Hormones During Menopause

Menopause is a natural phase in a woman's life when the ovaries produce less estrogen and progesterone, and menstrual cycles stop. It usually occurs in the late 40s to early 50s, but this can vary.

- **Symptoms**: Hot flashes, mood swings, sleep disturbances, and changes in body composition (often more belly fat).
- **Nutritional Focus**:
    - **Calcium and Vitamin D** to support bone health.
    - **Phytoestrogens** (found in soy foods like tofu, tempeh, edamame) may help some women manage mild hot flashes, though the research is mixed.
    - **Lean Protein and Strength Training** to help maintain muscle mass, which often declines with age.

5.13 The Gut-Hormone Connection

Your gut health can influence hormones, too. Certain bacteria in the gut help break down and eliminate excess hormones. If your gut microbiome is out of balance (perhaps due to too many processed foods, stress, or antibiotic use), it might affect how hormones circulate in your body.

- **Probiotics**: Found in yogurt, kefir, or fermented vegetables (kimchi, sauerkraut), might support a healthier gut.
- **Prebiotics**: Found in fiber-rich foods like onions, garlic, leeks, bananas, and oats, help feed beneficial gut bacteria.

5.14 Practical Steps to Support Hormonal Health

Let's summarize ways to keep hormones in balance:

1. **Eat Balanced Meals**: Include protein, carbs (preferably complex carbs like whole grains), and healthy fats in each meal.
2. **Choose Nutrient-Dense Foods**: Fruits, vegetables, whole grains, lean proteins, nuts, and seeds.
3. **Stay Hydrated**: Water is essential for many bodily processes, including the transport of hormones.
4. **Manage Stress**: Even short breaks, breathing exercises, or walks outside can lower cortisol.
5. **Prioritize Sleep**: Aim for 7–8 hours of quality sleep each night.
6. **Limit Ultra-Processed Foods**: They can cause spikes in insulin and might create inflammation, affecting hormone function.

5.15 Hormones and Cravings: A Real-Life Example

Imagine you have had a rough day at work. You feel stressed, and your energy is low. Your cortisol is up, and so is your hunger for quick-energy foods—maybe a donut or some ice cream. If this becomes a daily habit, it can lead to weight gain and potential blood sugar issues.

How to Cope:

- **Plan in advance**. If you know you get sugar cravings at night, keep healthier sweet options like frozen berries or dark chocolate squares.
- **Check your protein intake** during the day. Low protein can lead to blood sugar dips.
- **Try relaxation**: A five-minute stretch or a warm bath might help you wind down without turning to sugary snacks.

5.16 Emotional Well-being and Hormones

Hormones also play a role in mental and emotional health. Estrogen can influence serotonin, a neurotransmitter that affects mood. This is why some women experience mood swings during PMS or perimenopause. If mood issues become severe, like in Premenstrual Dysphoric Disorder (PMDD), it might require professional help or a more targeted approach, including possibly medication or therapy.

Nutrition can still be part of the puzzle: a balanced diet that supports stable blood sugar and includes mood-supporting nutrients (like omega-3 fats, magnesium, and B vitamins) can help ease some emotional ups and downs.

5.17 The Role of Blood Tests and Check-Ups

If you suspect hormone imbalances—irregular periods, unexplained weight gain or loss, extreme fatigue, mood issues—it could be wise to have a check-up with a healthcare professional. Blood tests can measure levels of thyroid hormones, insulin, cortisol, estrogen, progesterone, and more. Knowing your hormone status can guide your nutritional choices more effectively. For instance, if blood tests show low estrogen and bone density issues, you might focus more on calcium, vitamin D, and possibly phytoestrogens under medical guidance.

5.18 Combining Nutrition, Exercise, and Self-Care

No single factor works alone for hormonal balance. A "whole life" approach usually yields the best results:

1. **Exercise**: Helps burn excess glucose, improves insulin sensitivity, and reduces stress. Even a brisk 30-minute walk each day can help.
2. **Nutrition**: A well-rounded diet without too many processed carbs or added sugars will help keep insulin in check.
3. **Self-Care**: Mindfulness, journaling, or quiet hobbies can lower stress, thus reducing chronic cortisol elevation.
4. **Community and Support**: Having friends, family, or a support group can help you stay motivated and manage stress better, indirectly supporting healthier hormones.

5.19 Common Myths About Hormones and Nutrition

1. **"You Must Cut All Carbs to Fix Hormones."**
    - Not true. Complex carbohydrates in whole grains, beans, and vegetables can support stable blood sugar and provide important nutrients. The key is avoiding excessive refined carbs and sugar.
2. **"Soy Foods Always Cause Hormone Imbalances."**
    - While soy contains plant estrogens (phytoestrogens), moderate intake is generally safe for most women and may provide some benefits. If you have specific health concerns, talk to a doctor.
3. **"Only Older Women Need to Worry About Hormones."**
    - Hormone health matters at every age—teenagers, young adults, and women in midlife all have hormonal shifts that can affect well-being.

CHAPTER 6: REPRODUCTIVE HEALTH AND NUTRITION

6.1 Introduction to Reproductive Health

Reproductive health is about much more than just having children. It includes the menstrual cycle, fertility (the ability to conceive), hormonal balance, and even sexual well-being. Nutrition can play a supporting role in all these areas. For instance, certain nutrients can help regulate cycles, while others can support healthy pregnancies or ease symptoms of conditions like PCOS or endometriosis.

In earlier chapters, we explored the basics of nutrition, key nutrients, and hormones. Now we tie it together to see how food choices can influence the reproductive system, whether you plan to have children or not.

6.2 The Menstrual Cycle: Key Nutritional Needs

Every month (for most women of childbearing age), the body prepares for a possible pregnancy. The menstrual cycle has phases, each with shifting hormone levels:

- **Menstrual Phase**: The uterus sheds its lining, which causes bleeding.
- **Follicular Phase**: Follicles in the ovary grow. Estrogen rises.
- **Ovulation**: An egg is released, typically around day 14 in a 28-day cycle.
- **Luteal Phase**: Progesterone levels rise to prepare the uterus for implantation if fertilization occurs.

Nutritional Tips by Phase:

- **Menstrual Phase**: Focus on iron-rich foods (red meat, beans, spinach) to make up for blood loss.
- **Follicular Phase**: Estrogen rises. Keep your energy levels steady with balanced meals that include complex carbs and protein.
- **Ovulation**: Usually, your energy is higher. Continue to eat well-rounded meals, and include antioxidant-rich fruits and vegetables to support cell health.
- **Luteal Phase**: Progesterone is high, which can cause cravings or bloating. Include magnesium-rich foods (leafy greens, nuts) to help ease potential cramps and mood changes.

6.3 Preconception Nutrition

If you are planning to become pregnant, it is wise to pay attention to your diet well before conception. The nutrients you have stored in your body can affect early fetal development.

Key points for preconception nutrition:

1. **Folic Acid (Folate)**: Adequate intake (400–600 micrograms per day) lowers the risk of neural tube defects. Found in leafy greens, beans, fortified cereals.
2. **Healthy Weight**: Being underweight or overweight can affect ovulation and fertility. Aim for a balanced diet and moderate exercise to reach a weight that is healthy for you.
3. **Reduce Alcohol and Caffeine**: High amounts of caffeine (more than about 200 mg a day) might interfere with conception. Alcohol can harm fetal development even before you realize you are pregnant.
4. **Avoid High-Mercury Fish**: Mercury can be harmful to the baby's developing brain. Limit fish like swordfish, shark, and tilefish.

5. **General Nutrient Balance**: Ensure enough protein, iron, calcium, and essential fatty acids (like omega-3s).

6.4 Fertility Diet: Foods to Boost Fertility

While there is no guarantee that specific foods will instantly boost fertility, a balanced diet can help support your body's natural functions. Some researchers talk about a "fertility diet" emphasizing:

1. **Plant Proteins**: Beans, lentils, nuts, and seeds.
2. **Full-Fat Dairy** (in moderation): Some studies suggest that switching from low-fat to full-fat dairy may help some women ovulate more regularly, but this is not a hard rule.
3. **Complex Carbohydrates**: Whole grains, fruits, vegetables—foods that digest more slowly and keep insulin levels stable.
4. **Good Fats**: Avocado, nuts, seeds, and olive oil support hormone production.

Limiting trans fats (found in some processed and fried foods) is also recommended, as they can worsen insulin resistance and inflammation.

6.5 Nutrition for PCOS

Polycystic ovary syndrome (PCOS) is a common endocrine disorder among women of reproductive age. It is often associated with insulin resistance, high androgen levels, irregular periods, and ovarian cysts.

Diet Tips for PCOS:

- **Lower Glycemic Foods**: Foods that do not cause a big spike in blood sugar—whole grains, beans, vegetables, and fruits.
- **Adequate Protein**: Helps control appetite and supports stable blood sugar.

- **Healthy Fats**: Omega-3 fatty acids may help reduce inflammation.
- **Possible Supplements**: Some women benefit from inositol or vitamin D supplements, but consult a healthcare professional first.

Weight loss (if overweight) can improve hormone balance and insulin sensitivity, but the approach should be gradual and focused on sustainable lifestyle changes rather than crash diets.

6.6 PMS and PMDD: Easing Symptoms with Food

PMS (premenstrual syndrome) and **PMDD (premenstrual dysphoric disorder)** involve physical and emotional symptoms like bloating, mood swings, irritability, and fatigue. Nutrition can sometimes help reduce the severity of these symptoms.

- **Limit Salt**: Can reduce bloating and fluid retention.
- **Increase Magnesium**: Found in dark chocolate, spinach, and nuts; may help with mood and cramps.
- **Moderate Caffeine**: Excess caffeine can worsen anxiety and irritability.
- **Stay Hydrated**: Helps with bloating and can ease headaches.

If you have severe PMS or PMDD, talk to a healthcare professional. Lifestyle changes, therapy, or medication might be needed for more serious cases.

6.7 The Role of Weight in Reproductive Health

Being either severely underweight or overweight can disrupt hormones that regulate the menstrual cycle and ovulation. For instance, low body fat can lead to **amenorrhea** (absence of periods), while high body fat might contribute to insulin resistance, which can throw off hormone levels.

Healthy Body Fat Range: It varies by individual, but a moderate range is often considered around 21–33% for women, though athletes might have lower ranges, and others may feel healthier in slightly different ranges. The main goal is to maintain a weight that supports regular cycles and overall well-being.

6.8 Stress, Sleep, and Reproductive Health

Stress and lack of sleep can affect hormones like cortisol, which in turn can interfere with the normal functioning of the reproductive system. If you are struggling with irregular periods or fertility issues, consider looking at your stress levels and sleep quality.

- **Relaxation Techniques**: Yoga, gentle stretching, breathing exercises.
- **Set a Bedtime Routine**: Aim for 7–8 hours of sleep. Turn off screens 30 minutes before bed.
- **Avoid Stimulants**: Excess caffeine or heavy meals late at night might keep you awake and disturb hormonal rhythms.

6.9 Contraception and Nutrition

Many women use **birth control pills**, intrauterine devices (IUDs), or other hormonal methods to prevent pregnancy. Some forms of contraception may slightly affect nutrient needs or weight.

- **Oral Contraceptives**: Can sometimes affect levels of certain vitamins (like B vitamins) in the body, but the effect is usually small. If you have concerns, talk to a healthcare provider about testing or supplementation.
- **Hormonal IUD**: Typically acts locally in the uterus, so it may not have as big a nutritional impact as oral contraceptives.
- **Lifestyle and Diet**: Regardless of contraception method, continue to focus on balanced meals, regular exercise, and stress management for overall reproductive health.

6.10 Early Pregnancy: Key Nutritional Points

Once pregnant, the first trimester is vital for the baby's initial development. Some important points:

1. **Folic Acid (Folate)**: Helps prevent neural tube defects.
2. **Iron**: Supports the increased blood volume needed for you and the baby.
3. **Avoid Harmful Substances**: Alcohol, certain fish high in mercury, unpasteurized dairy, and raw or undercooked meats.
4. **Manage Nausea**: Some women experience morning sickness or food aversions. Eating small, frequent meals and bland foods (like crackers) can help.
5. **Stay Hydrated**: Water is essential, especially if you have nausea or vomiting.

6.11 Pregnancy Loss and Recovery (Including Miscarriage)

Sadly, not all pregnancies progress to term. If a woman experiences a miscarriage or other pregnancy loss, the body may need time to recover physically and emotionally.

- **Nutritional Needs**: Replenish iron if blood loss was significant. Focus on nutrient-rich foods like fruits, vegetables, lean proteins, and whole grains to support healing.
- **Emotional Support**: Grief, stress, or depression can affect appetite and overall health. Seek counseling or support groups if needed.

6.12 Postpartum Nutrition

After childbirth, a woman's body is healing, and if breastfeeding, she is providing nutrients for the baby as well:

1. **Extra Calories**: Breastfeeding can burn about 300–500 extra calories a day, but make those calories count with nutrient-dense foods.
2. **Protein and Calcium**: Supporting milk production and bone health.
3. **Hydration**: Essential for producing breast milk.
4. **Slow Weight Loss**: Many women want to "bounce back." Aim for gradual weight loss, as too much restriction can affect milk supply and energy levels.

6.13 The Importance of Consistency

Reproductive health is a long game. Your monthly cycles, fertility, and even menopause transitions depend on patterns of living. Trying a crash diet or quick fixes often does more harm than good. Instead, small, consistent improvements in your diet and lifestyle can lead to better menstrual regularity, improved fertility, and easier management of menopause symptoms.

6.14 Building a Support System

Women often juggle multiple roles—work, family, relationships—which can add stress and reduce the time available to plan healthy meals or exercise. Having a support system can make a big difference:

- **Family or Friends**: Maybe you can form a cooking club or share healthy recipes.
- **Healthcare Provider**: A doctor or nutritionist can give personalized advice, especially if you have a condition like PCOS or thyroid disease.
- **Online Communities**: Many women find tips, recipes, and encouragement through social media groups or forums focused on women's health.

6.15 Other Conditions Affecting Reproductive Health

1. **Endometriosis**: Tissue similar to the lining of the uterus grows outside of it, causing pain. Some women find relief with anti-inflammatory diets high in fruits, veggies, and omega-3 fats.
2. **Fibroids**: Non-cancerous tumors in the uterus. While diet alone might not cure fibroids, maintaining a healthy weight and reducing excess estrogen may help.
3. **Premature Ovarian Failure**: Early menopause, occurring before age 40. Nutrition with emphasis on calcium, vitamin D, and heart-healthy foods is important.

6.16 Sexual Health and Energy Levels

Nutrition can also impact libido and energy levels related to sexual well-being:

- **Blood Flow**: Foods that support heart health (like those rich in omega-3s, antioxidants, and fiber) can improve circulation.
- **Mood and Energy**: Iron and B vitamins can boost energy. Magnesium and vitamin D might help with mood regulation.
- **Hormone Production**: Adequate protein and healthy fats are needed for hormone creation.

6.17 Managing Cravings and Emotional Eating During Different Life Stages

Throughout a woman's reproductive life, cravings can pop up at many points—during PMS, pregnancy, postpartum stress, or even perimenopause. Being mindful of these cravings helps prevent going overboard:

- **Have Healthier Alternatives**: For sweet cravings, keep fruit or dark chocolate on hand. For salty cravings, try roasted chickpeas or lightly salted popcorn.

- **Plan Balanced Meals**: Protein, fiber, and healthy fats help stabilize blood sugar, reducing the likelihood of extreme cravings.
- **Identify Emotional Triggers**: Sometimes, cravings are tied to stress, boredom, or sadness rather than true hunger.

6.18 Contraceptive Transitions and Nutritional Shifts

Women might change contraceptive methods over time—switching from pills to an IUD or stopping birth control to try for a baby. Each transition can cause hormonal shifts that may influence weight, mood, or nutrient needs. Staying aware of these changes and adjusting your diet or supplement routine can help minimize unwanted effects like sudden weight changes or mood swings.

6.19 Health Check-Ups and Screenings

Regular check-ups are an important part of reproductive health. Pap smears, pelvic exams, and mammograms (for breast health) are recommended on a schedule advised by your doctor. Nutritional choices can support your overall health and might help reduce inflammation or maintain a healthy weight—both important for reducing the risk of certain cancers and complications.

CHAPTER 7: NUTRITION THROUGH DIFFERENT LIFE STAGES

7.1 Why Different Life Stages Matter for Women's Nutrition

Women's bodies go through many changes over a lifetime. Each stage—from young adolescence to post-menopause—brings different nutritional needs. When you understand these changes, you can make better choices to stay healthy and strong. For example, a teenage girl needs enough nutrients to support growth and bone development, while a woman in her 50s may need to focus more on maintaining muscle mass and preventing bone loss.

Our bodies are not static. Hormones, activity levels, and lifestyles shift as we get older. That is why learning about nutrition at each life stage can help you prepare for (and handle) these changes. Good nutrition is like a foundation that supports your body's changing structure and functions. Whether you are 15 or 65, the more you know, the more confident you will feel in caring for your health.

7.2 Adolescence (Ages ~10 to 18)

Key Concerns: Rapid growth, bone development, menstrual cycle onset, body image

1. **Calorie Needs and Growth**
   During puberty, girls have growth spurts, and their bodies start to build more bone mass. This requires extra calories and nutrients. If a teenage girl does not get enough of the right foods, she might miss out on reaching her full height potential or building strong bones for adulthood.

2. **Focus on Bone Health**
   The teen years are when bones absorb calcium at high rates, helping build a "bone bank" that can protect against osteoporosis later. Foods like low-fat dairy, calcium-fortified plant milks, leafy greens, and yogurt can give teens the calcium they need. Getting enough vitamin D (through safe sunlight exposure or fortified foods) also helps.
3. **Protein for Growth**
   Teens need protein to support muscle and tissue development. Good sources include lean meats, beans, nuts, seeds, eggs, and dairy. It can be helpful to include some protein at each meal—like peanut butter on whole grain toast or chicken in a sandwich.
4. **Healthy Fats and Brain Development**
   While the brain has already formed its basic structure by adolescence, it is still maturing. Omega-3 fatty acids (found in fish, walnuts, chia seeds) can support brain health during this stage.
5. **Handling Body Image**
   Adolescence can be a time of self-consciousness. Rapid body changes can lead to anxiety about weight or shape. Fad diets or severe calorie restriction can harm growth. Encourage balanced meals and remind teens their bodies are still developing.
6. **Iron for Menstruation**
   When menstruation begins, teenage girls lose some iron each month. Iron is essential for carrying oxygen in the blood. Lean meats, spinach, beans, and fortified cereals are good sources. Pairing these foods with vitamin C-rich foods (like oranges or tomatoes) can help the body absorb iron better.

7.3 Early Adulthood (Ages ~19 to 30)

Key Concerns: Busy schedules, building lifelong habits, possibly preparing for pregnancy

1. **Time Constraints**
   Many women in their 20s juggle school, new careers, or social lives. Quick meals and fast food can seem convenient. However, forming healthy habits now can set the tone for decades. Aim for "easy but healthy" meals like simple stir-fries, salads with protein, or sandwiches made with whole grain bread.
2. **Balanced Calories**
   Metabolism may still be relatively high in your early 20s, but it can slow slightly by your late 20s. Keeping an eye on portion sizes and balancing food groups helps prevent gradual weight gain.
3. **Maintaining Strong Bones**
   Peak bone mass is typically reached in your late 20s. Getting enough calcium and vitamin D remains important. Weight-bearing exercises like walking, running, or strength training help keep bones dense.
4. **Focusing on Key Nutrients**
   - **Folate (Folic Acid)**: Important if there's any chance of pregnancy, as it helps prevent certain birth defects.
   - **Protein**: Supports muscle maintenance, especially if you're physically active.
   - **Iron**: Helps avoid anemia, especially if monthly menstrual bleeding is heavy.
5. **Establishing Activity Routines**
   Regular exercise can be easier to maintain if started earlier in life. Activities can vary: gym workouts, dance classes, or sports teams. Any movement is better than none, and building a routine helps manage weight, stress, and energy levels.

7.4 The 30s: Balancing Career, Family, and Health

Key Concerns: Possible pregnancy, juggling responsibilities, preventing early metabolic slowdown

1. **Nutrient-Dense Choices**
   Many women in their 30s have busy careers, raising children, or both. This makes convenient foods tempting. Aim to pick nutrient-dense options whenever possible. Think brown rice or quinoa over white rice, grilled chicken instead of fried, or fresh fruit instead of candy.
2. **Pregnancy and Postpartum**
   If pregnancy is on the table, focus on a balanced intake of proteins, healthy fats, folate, iron, and calcium. If you've already gone through pregnancy and are in postpartum, remember that nutritional needs are still high if you are breastfeeding.
3. **Weight Management**
   Metabolism may slow more as you move through your 30s. It's normal to gain a little weight, but staying active and controlling portion sizes helps keep it in check. Strength training becomes more important in preserving muscle mass.
4. **Stress and Cortisol**
   With work, parenting, and other responsibilities, stress can spike cortisol levels. This can lead to cravings or emotional eating. Balancing meals and practicing stress management (like short walks or mindful breathing) can help.
5. **Monitoring Hormones**
   Subtle hormonal shifts can begin in some women's mid to late 30s. Being aware of changes (like irregular periods or lower energy) can help you adjust your diet by focusing on nutrient-rich foods and possibly discussing concerns with a healthcare provider.

7.5 The 40s: Shifting Toward Perimenopause

Key Concerns: Hormonal fluctuations, beginning of perimenopause, changes in body composition

1. **Perimenopause**
   Perimenopause is the transition phase leading up to

menopause. It can last for several years and is marked by fluctuating estrogen levels. Symptoms can include irregular periods, hot flashes, mood swings, and weight changes.

2. **Focus on Protein and Muscle Mass**
   Muscle mass gradually decreases with age, which can lower metabolism. Eating enough protein (and exercising with resistance training) helps preserve muscle. Good sources: poultry, fish, beans, lentils, eggs, dairy, tofu, or tempeh.

3. **Balancing Blood Sugar**
   Fluctuations in hormones can affect insulin sensitivity. Eating balanced meals with protein, fiber, and healthy fats keeps blood sugar steadier, reducing energy crashes or intense sugar cravings.

4. **Calcium and Vitamin D for Bones**
   Bone density may start to decline more noticeably in your 40s. Calcium, vitamin D, magnesium, and weight-bearing exercise remain crucial to help slow bone loss.

5. **Healthy Fats**
   Omega-3 fatty acids can help manage inflammation, which may rise with age. Include fish (like salmon or sardines) or plant-based sources (chia seeds, flaxseeds, walnuts) in your diet.

6. **Self-Care for Stress**
   Hormonal changes plus life stress (like caring for children, aging parents, or career demands) can be overwhelming. Remember that nutrition is part of self-care. Regular, balanced meals give your body the nutrients it needs to cope better with stress.

7.6 The 50s: Menopause and Beyond

Key Concerns: Lower estrogen, bone health, heart health, maintaining lean muscle

1. **Menopause Basics**
   Menopause is defined as going 12 months without a

menstrual period. During and after menopause, estrogen levels drop significantly, which can lead to an increased risk of osteoporosis and shifts in fat storage (often more around the abdomen).

2. **Bone Health**
Osteoporosis risk rises sharply after menopause. Meeting your calcium and vitamin D needs is vital. Foods like low-fat dairy, leafy greens, fortified plant milks, and vitamin D-rich fish can help. Some women may consider supplements if dietary intake is insufficient.

3. **Heart Health**
Estrogen helps protect against heart disease, so the risk goes up post-menopause. Focus on whole grains, fruits, vegetables, and lean proteins. Keep an eye on saturated fats and limit processed foods high in trans fats or added sugars.

4. **Managing Weight Gain**
With lower estrogen, metabolism can slow further. Smaller portions, regular exercise (including strength training), and mindful eating can help manage weight.

5. **Phytoestrogens**
Foods like soy (tofu, edamame, tempeh) contain plant estrogens that may help some women cope with mild menopause symptoms like hot flashes. However, effects can vary, and it is best to talk to a healthcare professional if you have questions, especially if you have a history of certain health conditions.

6. **Staying Hydrated**
Hot flashes can lead to extra sweating. Drinking enough water can prevent dehydration. Also, watch caffeine and alcohol, which can worsen hot flashes and night sweats.

7.7 Older Adulthood (60s, 70s, and Beyond)

Key Concerns: Maintaining muscle, preventing malnutrition, supporting cognitive health

1. **Appetite Changes**
   Sense of taste or smell might decrease with age. Some older adults lose interest in food or eat less, which can lead to nutrient gaps. Eating smaller, nutrient-dense meals throughout the day helps ensure enough protein, vitamins, and minerals.
2. **Protein to Prevent Muscle Loss**
   Sarcopenia (age-related muscle loss) can affect strength and mobility. Older women can benefit from slightly higher protein intake spread out over the day, paired with resistance exercises (light weights or bands).
3. **Easy-to-Chew Foods**
   Dental issues might make it hard to chew tough meats or raw vegetables. Soft cooked vegetables, ground meats, beans, and scrambled eggs can help. Smoothies with fruits, yogurt, and protein powder can be an option too.
4. **Hydration**
   Thirst signals can weaken in older age, leading to dehydration. It is important to sip water regularly, even if you do not feel particularly thirsty. Other beverages like low-sugar juices or herbal teas can also help.
5. **Micronutrients of Concern**
   - **Vitamin B12**: Absorption can decrease with age, so foods fortified with B12 or a supplement might be needed if blood tests show low levels.
   - **Calcium and Vitamin D**: Bone health continues to be crucial, especially to prevent fractures.
   - **Omega-3 Fats**: May help with joint health and possibly cognitive function.
6. **Preventing Isolation**
   Social factors can affect nutrition. Some older adults who live alone might lack motivation to cook. Sharing meals with friends, family, or community groups can help. Meal delivery services (like Meals on Wheels) may also be available.

7.8 Special Situations: Health Conditions and Medications

At any age, certain health conditions (like diabetes, high blood pressure, or thyroid issues) can influence nutritional needs. Some medications can also affect appetite or nutrient absorption. It is wise to:

- **Keep Healthcare Providers Informed**: Let them know about any diet changes or supplements.
- **Follow Up on Blood Tests**: Check for possible deficiencies in vitamin D, B12, or iron.
- **Adjust Diet as Needed**: If a doctor says to reduce sodium for high blood pressure, look for low-salt seasonings. If cholesterol is high, focus on fiber-rich foods and healthy fats.

CHAPTER 8: HEALTHY EATING PATTERNS AND MEAL PLANNING

8.1 Introduction to Eating Patterns

An **eating pattern** is the overall way you eat over time. It is not just one meal or one day of eating; it is the routine you follow on most days. Examples include the Mediterranean diet, the DASH diet (Dietary Approaches to Stop Hypertension), a plant-based diet, or simply a balanced "traditional" approach. The key is finding a pattern that provides your body with nutrients while fitting your preferences and lifestyle.

Meal planning is one strategy to keep you on track. When you plan your meals and snacks ahead of time, you are less likely to grab unhealthy options at the last minute. Instead, you choose foods that support your health goals—whether that is maintaining a stable weight, boosting energy, or getting enough vitamins and minerals.

8.2 Understanding Different Eating Patterns

While we will not repeat details from earlier chapters, let's highlight a few popular patterns and how they might fit into a woman's health goals.

1. **Mediterranean-Style Diet**
    - **Key Features**: High in fruits, vegetables, whole grains, legumes, fish, and healthy fats (like olive oil), with moderate dairy and limited red meat.
    - **Potential Benefits**: Good for heart health, may help manage weight, and could lower inflammation.
2. **DASH Diet (Dietary Approaches to Stop Hypertension)**

- **Key Features**: Emphasizes fruits, vegetables, whole grains, low-fat dairy, lean meats, and nuts. Focuses on reducing sodium to help control blood pressure.
- **Potential Benefits**: Helpful if you have high blood pressure or want a heart-friendly approach.

3. **Plant-Based Diet (Vegetarian or Vegan)**
   - **Key Features**: Focuses on fruits, vegetables, legumes, grains, nuts, and seeds, with no (or minimal) animal products.
   - **Potential Benefits**: Can be rich in fiber, vitamins, and antioxidants, but might need extra attention to nutrients like vitamin B12, iron, and protein.
4. **Flexitarian Diet**
   - **Key Features**: Primarily plant-based but includes small amounts of meat, fish, or poultry occasionally.
   - **Potential Benefits**: Offers the health perks of a plant-heavy diet while allowing animal products in moderation.
5. **Low-Carb or Moderate-Carb Plans**
   - **Key Features**: Reduces refined carbs (like white bread, pastries, sugary drinks) and focuses on proteins, healthy fats, and vegetables.
   - **Potential Benefits**: May help with weight management or blood sugar control, especially for women with insulin resistance or PCOS.

The best eating pattern is one you can sustain. Extreme diets or highly restrictive plans often fail because they are too hard to maintain in the long run. A balanced approach that includes a variety of foods typically leads to better health outcomes.

8.3 Building a Balanced Meal

No matter which eating pattern you choose, a balanced meal often includes:

1. **Protein**: Lean meats, fish, poultry, eggs, beans, tofu, or lentils.
2. **Complex Carbohydrates**: Whole grains (oats, brown rice, whole wheat pasta), starchy vegetables (sweet potatoes), or legumes.
3. **Non-Starchy Vegetables**: Broccoli, spinach, bell peppers, carrots, zucchini, etc.
4. **Healthy Fats**: Avocado, nuts, seeds, olive oil, or fatty fish.
5. **Optional Fruits**: A side of fresh fruit or a piece of fruit for dessert adds antioxidants, vitamins, and natural sweetness.

A quick way to visualize this is the **"plate method"**:

- Half of your plate: Vegetables or a mix of vegetables and fruits.
- One quarter: Protein.
- One quarter: Whole grains or complex carbohydrates.

8.4 Meal Planning Basics

Meal planning means deciding in advance what you will eat for breakfasts, lunches, dinners, and snacks. This can range from a simple list of meal ideas to a detailed schedule. The main benefits include:

- **Time Savings**: Having ingredients ready reduces last-minute fast-food trips.
- **Cost Savings**: Buying only what you plan to use can lower grocery bills.
- **Nutrient Control**: You can ensure each meal has a good balance of protein, carbs, and fats.
- **Less Food Waste**: If you stick to your plan, you are less likely to throw away unused items.

8.5 Step-by-Step Meal Planning

1. **Check Your Calendar**
   - Do you have busy days when you need a quick meal? Plan a fast recipe or leftovers for those days.
   - Any events, like dinners out or social gatherings, that mean you will not cook that night?
2. **Choose Your Recipes or Meal Types**
   - Pick a variety of proteins (chicken, fish, beans) and cuisines (Italian, Mexican, Asian) so you do not get bored.
   - Consider any special dietary needs (allergies, vegetarian choices, low-sodium if you have high blood pressure, etc.).
3. **Make a Grocery List**
   - List out every ingredient you need for the week. Check your pantry and fridge to avoid buying duplicates.
   - Organize the list by sections of the store (produce, dairy, meats) for faster shopping.
4. **Prep Ahead**
   - Wash and chop vegetables in advance.
   - Cook large batches of grains (like brown rice or quinoa) to use throughout the week.
   - Marinate meats or assemble slow-cooker ingredients the night before.
5. **Store Properly**
   - Use airtight containers, label items with dates, and keep a clear order in the fridge or freezer.
   - Put older items in front so they get used first.

8.6 Meal Prepping Strategies

Meal prep is slightly different from meal planning. It involves preparing parts of your meals (or entire meals) ahead of time to make actual cooking or assembling quicker. Here are a few methods:

1. **Batch Cooking**
   - Cook a big pot of soup, chili, or stew on the weekend. Portion into containers for lunches or quick dinners all week.
   - Cook large amounts of protein (like chicken breasts, ground turkey, or tofu) that can be used in salads, wraps, or stir-fries.
2. **Sheet Pan Meals**
   - Put protein (chicken, salmon, tofu) on a sheet pan with chopped veggies. Roast them all at once for a simple meal.
   - Make extra so you have leftovers for lunch.
3. **Freezer-Friendly Meals**
   - Certain dishes (like lasagna, casseroles, or veggie burgers) can be prepared in bulk and frozen. Then you can thaw and heat them when pressed for time.
4. **Grab-and-Go Snacks**
   - Wash and cut fruit. Portion them in small containers or bags.
   - Measure out trail mix or nuts. This prevents overeating and provides quick snacks.

The goal is to have healthy items ready so you are less tempted by fast food or junk snacks when hunger strikes.

8.7 Sample 7-Day Meal Plan

Below is a simple 7-day meal plan outline focusing on balanced meals. Feel free to adjust for portion sizes or dietary preferences. Note that this is just one example, not a strict prescription.

Day 1

- Breakfast: Oatmeal topped with berries and a drizzle of honey. Side of scrambled eggs for protein.
- Lunch: Whole grain tortilla wrap with turkey, lettuce, tomato, and a small amount of mayo or hummus. Side of carrot sticks.
- Dinner: Salmon fillet baked with lemon and herbs, brown rice, and steamed broccoli.
- Snack: Apple slices with peanut butter.

Day 2

- Breakfast: Yogurt parfait with low-fat yogurt, chopped strawberries, and granola.
- Lunch: Lentil soup (batch-cooked on the weekend), whole grain bread.
- Dinner: Chicken stir-fry with mixed vegetables (broccoli, peppers, onions) and a light sauce. Serve over quinoa.
- Snack: Cottage cheese with pineapple chunks.

Day 3

- Breakfast: Smoothie with spinach, banana, frozen berries, and a spoonful of peanut butter.
- Lunch: Tuna salad on whole grain crackers, side salad with mixed greens, cucumbers, and vinaigrette.
- Dinner: Veggie chili (beans, tomatoes, onions, peppers) topped with a sprinkle of cheese.
- Snack: Handful of almonds.

Day 4

- Breakfast: Whole grain toast with mashed avocado and a fried egg on top.
- Lunch: Baked sweet potato topped with black beans, salsa, and a dollop of Greek yogurt.
- Dinner: Turkey meatballs with marinara sauce, whole wheat pasta, and sautéed spinach.
- Snack: Banana with a small square of dark chocolate.

Day 5

- Breakfast: Egg white omelet with spinach and mushrooms, side of whole grain toast.
- Lunch: Chicken salad made with Greek yogurt, grapes, celery, served in a lettuce wrap.
- Dinner: Grilled shrimp or tofu skewers with bell peppers and onions, served over brown rice.
- Snack: Low-fat cheese stick and a handful of grapes.

Day 6

- Breakfast: Whole grain English muffin topped with peanut butter and sliced bananas.
- Lunch: Mixed green salad with grilled salmon (leftovers from earlier in the week), chickpeas, and a light dressing.
- Dinner: Homemade veggie pizza on whole wheat crust with tomato sauce, mozzarella cheese, and plenty of vegetables (like peppers, onions, mushrooms).
- Snack: Greek yogurt with honey and a sprinkle of cinnamon.

Day 7

- Breakfast: Whole grain pancakes with fresh berries. Go light on the syrup.
- Lunch: Minestrone soup (kidney beans, veggies, whole wheat pasta in a tomato broth).

- Dinner: Baked chicken breast, roasted zucchini, and a small baked potato with a little olive oil and herbs.
- Snack: Air-popped popcorn.

8.8 Adjusting for Dietary Needs and Preferences

- **Vegetarian/Vegan**: Replace meats and fish with beans, lentils, tofu, tempeh, or other plant proteins. Ensure adequate vitamin B12, iron, and protein intake.
- **Gluten-Free**: Swap whole wheat bread or pasta with certified gluten-free options like brown rice pasta, quinoa, or buckwheat noodles.
- **Low-Sodium**: Choose fresh over canned vegetables (or rinse canned ones), use herbs and spices instead of salt, and check labels for "low sodium" versions of broth or sauces.
- **Dairy-Free**: Use plant-based milks (almond, soy, oat) that are fortified with calcium and vitamin D. Swap yogurt or cheese with nondairy alternatives (just watch for added sugars).

8.9 Shopping Tips for Meal Planning

1. **Create a List and Stick to It**
   - Avoid impulse buys of snacks or sweets you do not actually need.
2. **Shop the Perimeter**
   - Most grocery stores keep produce, meats, dairy, and whole foods around the outer edges. The center aisles often have processed products.
3. **Buy in Bulk (for Some Items)**
   - Items like beans, lentils, brown rice, oats, and nuts can be cheaper when bought in bulk. Store them properly to keep them fresh.
4. **Compare Unit Prices**
   - Check the cost per ounce or per gram. Sometimes, bigger packages are cheaper overall.
5. **Choose Seasonal Produce**

- Fruits and vegetables in season often taste better and cost less. Frozen produce can also be a good choice if fresh options are out of season or more expensive.

8.10 Eating Out While Sticking to a Plan

Meal planning does not mean you cannot enjoy restaurants or social events. It just helps you make better choices when you do:

- **Check the Menu Ahead**
    - Many restaurants post menus online. Look for grilled or baked items, vegetable sides, and avoid heavy cream sauces.
- **Portion Control**
    - Restaurant servings can be large. Consider sharing a dish or asking for a to-go box right away.
- **Go Easy on Sugary Drinks**
    - Sugary sodas, specialty coffees, and cocktails can add many extra calories and sugars. Water, unsweetened tea, or sparkling water are alternatives.

8.11 Handling Cravings and Emotional Eating

Even with the best meal plan, cravings can strike. Emotional eating can derail healthy patterns if you are not prepared:

- **Identify Triggers**
    - Are you stressed, bored, or sad? Sometimes cravings are about emotions, not actual hunger.
- **Have Substitutes Ready**
    - If you crave sweets, keep fruit or a small piece of dark chocolate on hand. If you want salty chips, try whole grain crackers with hummus.
- **Mindful Eating**

- Take a moment to breathe before you eat. Ask yourself if you are truly hungry or just feeling an emotional need.

8.12 Budget-Friendly Meal Planning

1. **Cook More at Home**
   - Restaurant meals cost more. Simple home-cooked meals can be both cheaper and healthier.
2. **Use Leftovers**
   - Turn leftover chicken into a sandwich or leftover veggies into a soup. This reduces waste and saves money.
3. **Embrace Simple Recipes**
   - Fancy recipes with many ingredients can get pricey. Basic meals with fewer ingredients can still be tasty and nutritious.
4. **Limit High-Cost Proteins**
   - Reducing red meat intake and using more beans or lentils can lower grocery bills while improving health.

8.13 Time-Saving Tips for Meal Preparation

1. **Use a Slow Cooker or Instant Pot**
   - Throw ingredients in before work, and dinner is ready when you get home.
2. **Double Up**
   - Whenever you cook, make double or triple and freeze the extra.
3. **Make It a Family Activity**
   - If you have kids, let them help wash vegetables or measure ingredients. This not only saves time but teaches them about healthy cooking.

8.14 Staying Flexible

Life happens, and sometimes your meal plan may not go as expected. Maybe you have to work late or you are missing an ingredient:

- **Have Backup Meals**
    - Keep a few quick, healthy items on hand, such as frozen veggies, canned beans, whole grain pasta, and ready-to-eat sauces.
- **Allow for Swaps**
    - If you planned salmon but the store does not have fresh salmon, pick another lean protein like chicken or a vegetarian option.

8.15 Mindful Meal Planning for Various Life Stages

As discussed in Chapter 7, women's nutritional needs vary by age. Adjust your meal planning accordingly:

- **Teens**: Focus on calcium-rich meals and snacks to support bone growth. Keep healthy, grab-and-go foods on hand to match a teen's active schedule.
- **Pregnancy**: Include folate-rich foods (leafy greens, beans), iron sources, and balanced meals to support the increased nutritional demands.
- **Postpartum and Breastfeeding**: Consider adding snacks high in protein or complex carbs to support milk production.
- **Menopause and Beyond**: Plan meals that feature calcium, vitamin D, and protein to fight muscle loss and bone density decline.

8.16 Technology for Meal Planning

Many apps can help you:

- **Track Grocery Lists**
- **Suggest Recipes** based on ingredients you already have
- **Scan Barcodes** to see nutritional details
- **Plan Weekly Menus** and even automatically generate shopping lists

Pick an app that feels easy to use. If you prefer pen and paper, a simple notebook or printed planner works fine, too.

8.17 Common Pitfalls in Meal Planning

1. **Overly Ambitious Plans**
   - Planning complicated recipes every day can lead to burnout. Keep it simple.
2. **Forgetting Snacks**
   - If you skip planning for snacks, you might grab unhealthy items out of hunger.
3. **Not Being Realistic**
   - Be honest about how much time you have to cook. If your week is hectic, opt for quick-cook meals or batch cooking.
4. **No Variety**
   - Eating the same meals every week can cause boredom. Try rotating new recipes or seasonal ingredients.

8.18 Making Meal Planning a Habit

Habits form when you repeat actions until they feel natural. Try these steps:

1. **Set Aside Time**
   - Pick one day a week (often a weekend) to plan meals, shop, and maybe do some meal prep.
2. **Stay Organized**

- Keep favorite recipes in one place—whether that is a recipe box, bookmarks on your phone, or a folder on your computer.
3. **Reflect and Adjust**
    - At the end of each week, see what worked and what did not. Adjust your plan to reduce waste or to fit your schedule better next time.

8.19 The Connection Between Meal Planning and Mental Health

When you plan meals:

- You reduce day-to-day stress about what to cook.
- You feel more in control of your health choices.
- You might save money, which can ease financial stress.
- You often free up more time for other activities or for rest.

Having a calmer, more organized approach to eating can support emotional well-being. It may also reduce the likelihood of emotional eating since you have set meals ready.

CHAPTER 9: SPECIAL DIETS AND FOOD CHOICES

9.1 Introduction to Special Diets

In earlier chapters, we covered general nutrition principles and how to plan balanced meals. But many people follow specific diets for health, ethical, or personal reasons. A **special diet** is any eating plan that has specific rules or excludes (or emphasizes) certain foods. Examples include vegetarian or vegan diets, gluten-free diets, and low-carb or paleo plans. Sometimes these choices are driven by allergies, medical conditions (like celiac disease), ethical beliefs, or the desire to achieve particular health outcomes.

Women often turn to special diets to manage weight, address hormonal issues, or improve energy levels. Some diets might help with certain health goals, but they can also have risks if not followed carefully. For instance, removing major food groups might lead to nutrient gaps. In this chapter, we will explore several common special diets, discuss possible benefits and drawbacks, and look at ways women can make healthy food choices within any chosen eating pattern.

9.2 Vegetarian and Vegan Diets

Vegetarian diets exclude meat, poultry, and fish, but may include eggs and dairy (depending on the exact type). **Vegan** diets exclude all animal products, including eggs, dairy, and often honey.

9.2.1 Why Some Women Choose Vegetarian or Vegan

1. **Ethical Reasons**: Concern for animal welfare or the environment.

2. **Health Benefits**: Lower intake of saturated fats from red meats, higher intake of fruits and vegetables.
3. **Religious or Cultural Practices**: Some traditions encourage vegetarianism or limit meat consumption.

9.2.2 Possible Health Advantages

- **High Fiber**: Plant-based diets often include more beans, fruits, and vegetables. These contain beneficial fiber and help with digestion.
- **Rich in Micronutrients**: Vegetables, fruits, nuts, and seeds can be high in vitamins, minerals, and antioxidants that support overall health.
- **Lower Saturated Fat**: Skipping or minimizing red meat reduces saturated fat intake, potentially helping heart health.

9.2.3 Potential Challenges for Women

- **Protein Intake**: While beans, lentils, tofu, and nuts contain protein, planning is needed to ensure adequate amounts, especially for women who are pregnant, breastfeeding, or very active.
- **Iron Levels**: Plant-based (non-heme) iron is harder for the body to absorb than heme iron from animal sources. Women who lose iron through menstruation need to be mindful. Pairing iron-rich foods (spinach, beans) with vitamin C–rich foods (citrus fruits) can boost absorption.
- **Vitamin B12**: This vitamin is mostly found in animal foods. Vegans especially may need B12-fortified products (like certain plant milks or cereals) or a supplement.
- **Calcium and Vitamin D**: If dairy is avoided, women must find fortified plant milks or other sources to support bone health.

9.2.4 Tips for Success

- **Variety**: Incorporate beans, lentils, tofu, tempeh, nuts, and seeds for protein.

- **Fortified Foods**: Choose cereals, plant milks, and nutritional yeast that contain B12, vitamin D, and calcium.
- **Meal Planning**: Combine complementary proteins (like rice and beans) to get all essential amino acids.
- **Regular Check-Ups**: Monitor iron levels and B12 levels with blood tests if you suspect a deficiency.

9.3 Gluten-Free Diets

A **gluten-free** diet excludes gluten, a protein found in wheat, barley, and rye. People with **celiac disease** must avoid gluten to prevent damage to their intestines. Others may have **non-celiac gluten sensitivity**, where gluten triggers uncomfortable symptoms like bloating or fatigue.

9.3.1 Reasons Women Go Gluten-Free

- **Medical Necessity**: Celiac disease or a diagnosed gluten intolerance.
- **Suspected Sensitivity**: Some women may experience better digestion or reduced bloating when cutting out gluten.
- **Health Trend**: A belief that gluten-free is "healthier" for everyone, which is not necessarily true unless there is a genuine intolerance.

9.3.2 Benefits and Drawbacks

- **Benefits**:
    - Essential for celiac patients to prevent intestinal damage, malnutrition, and other serious complications.
    - Might improve digestive symptoms (bloating, diarrhea) for those who are truly sensitive.
- **Drawbacks**:
    - Restrictive: Avoiding wheat, barley, rye, and many common processed foods can be challenging.

- Nutrient Gaps: Many gluten-free products are lower in fiber and certain vitamins unless they are fortified.
- Cost: Gluten-free specialty items can be more expensive.

9.3.3 Helpful Tips

- **Focus on Whole Foods**: Naturally gluten-free grains include rice, quinoa, buckwheat, corn, and millet.
- **Read Labels Carefully**: Gluten hides in sauces, processed meats, soups, and more.
- **Fortify and Supplement**: If you rely heavily on gluten-free packaged foods, ensure you get enough fiber, B vitamins, and iron from other sources.

9.4 Low-Carb, Keto, and Paleo Diets

In recent years, low-carb and high-fat diets have become popular for weight management and other possible health benefits. Let's look at three well-known approaches.

9.4.1 Low-Carb Diets

- **Definition**: Typically limit carbohydrate intake to less than about 40% of daily calories. Some variations are stricter.
- **Common Foods**: Meat, fish, eggs, non-starchy vegetables, nuts, seeds, and limited fruit.
- **Pros**: May help some women reduce insulin spikes, manage blood sugar, or lose weight in the short term.
- **Cons**: If not planned properly, low-carb diets can lack fiber and important nutrients found in whole grains, fruits, and legumes.

9.4.2 Ketogenic (Keto) Diet

- **Definition**: Ultra-low carb (usually under 20–50 grams of carbs per day), high fat, moderate protein. The goal is to enter **ketosis**, where the body burns fat for fuel.
- **Pros**: Some people report quick weight loss, better blood sugar control, or reduced appetite.
- **Cons**:
    - Restrictive: Severely limiting carbs means cutting out most fruits, many vegetables, and grains.
    - Nutrient Gaps: Risk of low intake of certain vitamins, minerals, or fiber.
    - May Not Suit Everyone: Women with thyroid issues, pregnant women, or those with certain hormonal imbalances should be cautious.

9.4.3 Paleo Diet

- **Definition**: Focuses on foods presumed to have been eaten by early humans—meat, fish, fruits, vegetables, nuts, seeds—while excluding dairy, grains, legumes, and refined sugar.
- **Pros**: Emphasizes whole foods, can reduce intake of processed junk foods.
- **Cons**:
    - Restrictive: Excludes whole grains and legumes, which are nutritious and beneficial for many women.
    - Potential Calcium Deficit: Cutting out dairy may lower calcium unless you rely on vegetables or supplements.

9.5 Intermittent Fasting

Intermittent fasting (IF) is not about what you eat, but when you eat. Common methods include:

- **16:8 Method**: Fast for 16 hours, eat within an 8-hour window each day.
- **5:2 Diet**: Eat normally for 5 days of the week, and severely restrict calories (e.g., 500–600 calories) for 2 days.

9.5.1 Possible Benefits

- **Weight Management**: Some people naturally reduce overall calorie intake when eating only in a limited time window.
- **Insulin Sensitivity**: Fasting periods may help stabilize blood sugar.
- **Simplicity**: Some find it easier to follow a schedule rather than tracking every calorie.

9.5.2 Concerns for Women

- **Hormonal Disruption**: Women's bodies can be sensitive to changes in eating patterns. Fasting might affect menstruation or fertility if it becomes too extreme.
- **Risk of Overeating**: Restricting too long can lead to bingeing when the eating window opens.
- **Stress**: Fasting can increase cortisol levels in some individuals. If you already have high stress, it might not help.

9.5.3 Tips for Safe Practice

- **Ease In**: Start with a 12-hour overnight fast (e.g., stop eating at 7 PM, resume at 7 AM). See how your body reacts.
- **Stay Hydrated**: Drink water, herbal tea, or other non-caloric beverages during fasting.
- **Listen to Your Body**: If you feel faint, overly stressed, or have disruptions in your menstrual cycle, consider modifying or stopping IF.

9.6 Potential Pitfalls and Myths About Special Diets

1. "One Size Fits All"

- Myth: A diet that works for your friend will work exactly the same for you. In reality, genetics, lifestyle, hormones, and preferences differ widely.
2. **"Carbs Are Evil"**
   - Myth: While too many refined carbs can be harmful, complex carbs like whole grains and beans provide valuable nutrients and fiber.
3. **"Going Gluten-Free Always Means Healthier"**
   - Myth: Gluten-free processed foods can still be high in sugar or unhealthy fats.
4. **"I Can Load Up on Processed Vegan Junk Food"**
   - Myth: Vegan diets can be healthy, but eating lots of potato chips, fries, or sugary vegan desserts can lead to weight gain and nutrient deficiencies.
5. **"High-Protein Means Unlimited Bacon"**
   - Myth: A balanced high-protein diet still needs lean protein sources, veggies, and healthy fats. Loading up on processed meats high in sodium and saturated fat can harm heart health.

9.7 Considering Individual Health Conditions

- **PCOS**: Women with PCOS may benefit from lower-carb diets or focusing on whole foods to improve insulin sensitivity. But extremely low-carb diets may disrupt hormones if taken too far.
- **Endometriosis**: An anti-inflammatory approach—rich in fruits, vegetables, omega-3 fats—may help reduce pain.
- **Thyroid Issues**: Very restrictive diets might not be ideal if you have hypothyroidism or hyperthyroidism. Consult a doctor or dietitian.
- **Pregnancy**: Special diets should be approached cautiously during pregnancy. Certain diets (like strict keto) can reduce essential nutrients for fetal growth.

9.8 Combining Diets and Personalizing Your Approach

Some people choose a **hybrid approach**—for instance, a mostly plant-based diet that occasionally includes fish (a pescatarian approach) or a Mediterranean-style plan that reduces gluten if they suspect sensitivity. The key is to make sure you are meeting nutritional needs:

1. **Check Macronutrients**: Protein, carbs, and fats in proportions that suit your energy and health requirements.
2. **Mind Micronutrients**: If you cut out entire food groups, where will you get calcium, iron, or vitamin D?
3. **Listen to Your Body**: If a diet leaves you feeling sluggish or causes irregular periods, it may not be the right fit.

9.9 Social and Practical Factors

- **Eating Out**: Special diets might limit menu choices. You may need to check restaurant menus in advance or ask for substitutions.
- **Family and Cultural Traditions**: Some dietary changes can conflict with traditional meal patterns. It may take creativity to adapt.
- **Expense and Availability**: Specialty products (like gluten-free flours, vegan cheeses, or organic grass-fed meats) can be costly. Consider budget-friendly alternatives like beans, lentils, frozen vegetables, and in-season produce.

CHAPTER 10: MANAGING WEIGHT IN A HEALTHY WAY

10.1 Understanding Weight Management

In society, there is often a strong focus on women's body weight and shape. This can lead to confusion and unhealthy behaviors if not approached with the right mindset. **Weight management** means finding and maintaining a weight that supports overall health, energy, and quality of life. It is not about being extremely thin or conforming to a single beauty standard.

Your healthy weight depends on multiple factors: body composition (the ratio of fat to muscle), age, genetics, medical conditions, and personal preferences. In this chapter, we will explore strategies for managing weight in a balanced way, avoiding crash diets, and paying attention to the emotional aspects of eating.

10.2 The Basics: Calories and Energy Balance

Energy balance is the relationship between the calories you consume through food and drink and the calories your body burns through basic functions (like breathing, circulation) and physical activity.

- **Calorie Deficit**: Eating fewer calories than you burn leads to weight loss over time.
- **Calorie Surplus**: Eating more calories than you burn can cause weight gain.
- **Calorie Maintenance**: Eating roughly the same amount you burn keeps weight stable.

While the basic formula of "calories in vs. calories out" matters, it is not the only factor. Hormones, metabolism, and the types of foods you eat also play significant roles.

10.3 Why Fad Diets Often Fail

1. **Too Restrictive**: Many crash diets cut calories or entire food groups drastically. This can cause nutrient deficiencies and a rebound effect once you return to normal eating.
2. **Unsustainable**: If a diet is too rigid or unrealistic, it is hard to follow long-term.
3. **Muscle Loss**: Severe calorie restriction can lead to losing muscle along with fat, lowering your metabolic rate.
4. **Psychological Stress**: Constantly feeling deprived can increase stress and the likelihood of overeating or bingeing.

A healthier approach looks at gradual changes, portion control, and balanced meals that you can maintain over time.

10.4 Setting Realistic Goals

When trying to manage weight, it helps to have **specific, measurable, achievable** goals:

- **Aim for Slow and Steady**: 1–2 pounds (about 0.5–1 kg) of weight loss per week is a common guideline for sustainability, though this varies by individual.
- **Non-Scale Goals**: Instead of only focusing on the number on the scale, look for improvements in energy, mood, or fitness.
- **Address Underlying Issues**: If emotional eating or stress is driving weight gain, tackle those issues directly rather than relying solely on diet changes.

10.5 Balancing Macronutrients

While we talked about special diets in Chapter 9, you do not have to follow a strict approach to manage weight. A balanced diet that includes **protein, complex carbohydrates, and healthy fats** can help you feel full and satisfied without overeating.

- **Protein**: Helps preserve muscle mass, which is crucial for a healthy metabolism.
- **Complex Carbs**: Provide steady energy and often include fiber (whole grains, beans, vegetables).
- **Healthy Fats**: Support hormone function and absorb certain vitamins (avocados, nuts, seeds, olive oil).

10.6 The Role of Exercise

Physical activity is a key component of weight management, offering numerous benefits beyond just burning calories:

1. **Muscle Preservation and Building**: Resistance training (weights, resistance bands) helps maintain or increase muscle mass, which burns more calories at rest than fat does.
2. **Cardiovascular Health**: Activities like walking, running, cycling, and swimming improve heart and lung health, also aiding in weight control.
3. **Stress Relief**: Exercise releases endorphins, which can reduce stress and emotional eating.
4. **Bone Health**: Weight-bearing exercises help keep bones strong—crucial for women, especially later in life.

Even short bursts of movement (like brisk walks) throughout the day can add up. The key is to find activities you enjoy so you will stick with them.

10.7 Mindful Eating for Weight Control

Mindful eating means paying close attention to what, when, and why you are eating. It can help you recognize true hunger versus emotional or boredom-driven eating.

- **Eat Without Distractions**: Turn off the TV, put away your phone, and really focus on the flavors, textures, and smells of your food.
- **Assess Hunger Levels**: Ask yourself how hungry you are before you eat. Are you physically hungry or just stressed or bored?
- **Slow Down**: It takes about 20 minutes for your brain to register fullness. Putting your fork down between bites and chewing thoroughly can prevent overeating.
- **Stop When Satisfied**: Aim to feel content, not stuffed.

10.8 Emotional Eating and Stress Management

Stress, sadness, or even happiness can trigger overeating if you use food as a coping mechanism. Learning healthier ways to handle emotions is key:

- **Identify Triggers**: Keep a journal of your mood and eating habits. Notice patterns—like reaching for sugary snacks when deadlines approach.
- **Find Alternatives**: If you are feeling overwhelmed, go for a short walk, call a friend, or do deep breathing exercises instead of eating mindlessly.
- **Seek Support**: If emotional eating is severe or linked to deeper issues (anxiety, depression), a counselor or therapist can help you develop better coping strategies.

10.9 Approaches to Healthy Weight Loss

1. **Portion Control**
   - Use smaller plates.
   - Measure servings until you learn to estimate properly.
   - Fill up on vegetables and salads first.
2. **Increase Protein and Fiber**
   - Protein (lean meats, beans, tofu) and fiber (vegetables, fruits, whole grains) both increase satiety.
3. **Cut Back on Added Sugars**
   - Sugary drinks, desserts, and candies provide calories with little nutritional value.
4. **Choose Nutrient-Dense Foods**
   - Focus on whole grains, lean proteins, fruits, vegetables, and healthy fats. Avoid empty calories like chips, soda, and sugary cereals.
5. **Include Physical Activity**
   - Aim for at least 150 minutes of moderate-intensity exercise per week, plus strength training sessions.
6. **Stay Hydrated**
   - Sometimes thirst is mistaken for hunger. Drinking enough water can help regulate appetite.

10.10 Approaches to Healthy Weight Gain

Some women may struggle to gain weight or maintain a higher weight due to high metabolism, certain medical conditions, or other factors.

- **Increase Caloric Density**: Add healthy fats (avocado, nut butter) to meals. Snack on nuts or trail mix.
- **Eat More Frequently**: Six smaller meals a day might be easier than three large ones.
- **Strength Training**: Building muscle is a key part of gaining healthy weight.

- **Choose Nutrient-Dense Foods**: Do not just load up on junk food; aim for quality calories like whole grains, lean protein, and healthy fats.

10.11 Keeping a Positive Body Image

Body image issues can develop if weight management goals become obsessive. You can care for your health while also practicing self-acceptance:

1. **Focus on Health Indicators**: Are you sleeping well? Do you have good energy levels? Can you engage in activities you enjoy?
2. **Avoid Constant Comparison**: Everyone's body type is different. Comparing yourself to others (including social media images) can fuel negative thoughts.
3. **Celebrate Non-Physical Traits**: Reflect on your kindness, intelligence, or sense of humor—there's more to you than your weight.
4. **Look for Support**: Friends, family, or professional counselors can help you maintain a healthy perspective.

10.12 Dealing with Plateaus

Weight plateaus are common. You might lose weight steadily at first, then suddenly no change occurs. This can happen due to the body adjusting to lower caloric intake or a specific activity level.

- **Reevaluate Your Calorie Needs**: As you lose weight, your body needs fewer calories.
- **Vary Your Workouts**: Challenge your muscles in new ways—try interval training, heavier weights, or a different cardio activity.
- **Track More Accurately**: Sometimes small extras (like sauces, condiments, or mindless snacking) slip in unnoticed. Logging food for a short period might help identify hidden calories.

- **Stay Patient**: Weight loss is not a straight line. Minor fluctuations or periods of no change are normal.

10.13 Weight Management During Different Life Stages

As we discussed in Chapter 7, women's bodies shift during adolescence, pregnancy, menopause, and older adulthood. Here's how weight management ties in:

- **Teens**: Avoid drastic diets that can disrupt growth. Focus on balanced meals to support bone development.
- **Pregnancy**: Weight gain is normal and needed for a healthy pregnancy. Restrictive diets are risky without medical guidance.
- **Postpartum**: It often takes time to lose baby weight. Caring for a newborn can be stressful—kindness to yourself is crucial.
- **Menopause**: Hormonal changes can slow metabolism. Adjust portion sizes and maintain muscle with strength training.

10.14 Supplements and Weight Management

There are countless "fat burner" or "weight loss" supplements on the market. Most of these lack solid scientific backing and might have side effects. Supplements that **may** have some limited support include:

- **Protein Powders**: Helpful if you struggle to meet protein needs through whole foods.
- **Fiber Supplements**: Could help with fullness if your diet is low in fiber.
- **Multivitamins**: Might fill small nutrient gaps but do not directly cause weight loss.

Always talk to a healthcare professional before trying any supplement, especially if you have underlying medical conditions.

10.15 Technology and Tools

Many women use apps or devices to track activity and calorie intake. Examples include:

- **Fitness Trackers (Wearables)**: Count steps, monitor heart rate, and estimate calories burned.
- **Food Tracking Apps**: MyFitnessPal, Cronometer, or others let you log meals and watch macro or micronutrient levels.
- **Smart Scales**: Measure weight, estimate body fat percentage, and track trends over time.

While these tools can be helpful, avoid becoming overly fixated on numbers. The main point is to gain awareness, not obsess over every detail.

10.16 Social Support and Accountability

Weight management can be easier with friends or family on board:

- **Workout Buddies**: Exercise with a friend to stay motivated.
- **Healthy Meal Swaps**: Host potlucks or recipe exchanges.
- **Online Communities**: Join supportive forums, but be wary of advice that promotes extreme dieting.

10.17 Professional Help

If you have tried multiple methods without success or if you suspect an eating disorder, consider seeking professional help:

- **Registered Dietitians**: Can create a personalized meal plan and address nutritional gaps.
- **Therapists or Counselors**: Can help tackle emotional or psychological issues related to weight and body image.
- **Doctors**: May run tests to see if medical conditions (like thyroid disorders) are affecting weight.

10.18 Maintaining Weight Loss

Research suggests many people regain lost weight within a year or two. To keep it off:

- **Keep Up the Habits**: Do not go back to old eating patterns. Continue portion control, choosing nutrient-dense foods, and staying active.
- **Adjust Goals as Needed**: If your lifestyle or preferences change, tweak your eating and exercise routines accordingly.
- **Stay Aware of Behaviors**: Occasional weigh-ins, food journaling, or self-checks can catch small weight gains before they become large.
- **Allow Flexibility**: Occasional treats or "off plan" meals are fine. The key is balance over time.

10.19 Special Situations

1. **PCOS**: Women with PCOS may find it tougher to lose weight due to insulin resistance. A diet lower in refined carbs, along with strength training, can help.
2. **Hypothyroidism**: Can slow metabolism. Proper medication, consistent exercise, and patience are important.
3. **Recovery from Disordered Eating**: Weight management may need a structured approach guided by mental health professionals to avoid relapse.

CHAPTER 11: ENERGY, PERFORMANCE, AND EXERCISE

11.1 Why Energy and Performance Matter for Women

Whether you are a casual walker, a recreational sports enthusiast, or a serious athlete, proper nutrition plays a big part in your energy levels and performance. Women sometimes face unique challenges, like juggling busy schedules, managing monthly hormonal changes, or dealing with social pressure about body size. By fueling your body correctly, you can get the most out of your workouts, stay strong, and reduce the risk of injury.

This chapter focuses on how to support your energy needs before, during, and after exercise. We will look at the roles of carbohydrates, proteins, fats, vitamins, and minerals, as well as cover hydration and the impact of overtraining or underfueling. You will see that exercise is not just for weight management; it can help improve mood, strengthen bones, maintain muscle, and boost overall health.

11.2 How the Body Produces Energy

Energy for physical activity comes from the calories in the food you eat. Your body can draw on different "fuel tanks," depending on the intensity and length of the activity:

1. **Immediate Energy (ATP-PC System)**
    - This system uses adenosine triphosphate (ATP) and phosphocreatine (PC) stored in muscles. It provides short bursts of power for a few seconds (like sprinting or jumping).

- It does not use oxygen or require complex chemical pathways. However, it runs out quickly.
2. **Anaerobic Glycolysis**
    - When you do moderately intense exercise (like a fast run) for up to about two minutes, your body breaks down glucose (carbohydrates) without much oxygen.
    - This method produces energy more slowly than the ATP-PC system but can last a little longer. It also creates lactate as a byproduct, which can lead to muscle fatigue if it builds up.
3. **Aerobic System**
    - For longer activities (like jogging, cycling, or swimming for many minutes), your body relies on aerobic metabolism, which requires oxygen to break down carbohydrates and fats.
    - This system is sustainable for a longer period, though it is not as explosive as anaerobic systems.

11.3 The Role of Carbohydrates, Proteins, and Fats

For women seeking to maximize performance, knowing how much of each macronutrient to consume is key.

1. **Carbohydrates**
    - Primary fuel source, especially for moderate to high-intensity exercise.
    - Stored in muscles and the liver as glycogen. Having enough glycogen can delay fatigue and improve endurance.
    - Complex carbs (whole grains, beans, vegetables) generally offer more vitamins, minerals, and fiber than refined carbs.
2. **Proteins**
    - Helps repair and build muscle. Essential for recovery after exercise.

- Can be used as an energy source if carb intake is too low, but that is not ideal since protein is better for tissue repair.
- Lean meats, fish, eggs, beans, dairy, soy products, nuts, and seeds are common protein sources.

3. **Fats**
    - Important for long-duration, lower-intensity activities (like walking, easy cycling, or casual hiking).
    - Necessary for hormone production and vitamin absorption.
    - Focus on unsaturated fats (avocados, nuts, seeds, olive oil) instead of high levels of saturated or trans fats.

11.4 Fueling for Different Types of Workouts

1. **Strength Training** (weightlifting, resistance exercises)
    - Goals: Build or maintain muscle, improve strength.
    - Suggested Fuel:
        - Enough protein to support muscle repair (around 20–30 grams of protein per meal, though needs vary).
        - Moderate carbs for energy.
        - Healthy fats for overall health.
2. **Endurance Training** (running, cycling, swimming)
    - Goals: Sustain energy over a longer period, delay fatigue.
    - Suggested Fuel:
        - Emphasize carbs (both before and possibly during very long events).
        - Adequate protein for muscle repair and maintenance.
        - Do not neglect healthy fats, but the main focus for long events is carbohydrate availability.
3. **High-Intensity Interval Training (HIIT)**

- Goals: Short bursts of intense effort followed by periods of rest.
- Suggested Fuel:
  - A balanced intake of carbs and protein is beneficial.
  - Carbs help power those sprints or explosive moves.
  - Protein supports muscle recovery, especially important if workouts are frequent.

11.5 Pre-Workout Nutrition

Eating the right foods before exercise can help you perform better and reduce the chance of fatigue:

1. **Timing**: Aim to have a balanced meal or snack 1–3 hours before working out. A meal closer to 3 hours before might include more substantial foods. If you are eating 1 hour before, keep it lighter.
2. **What to Eat**:
   - **Carbs**: Provide quick energy. Examples: oatmeal, whole grain toast, fruit, or a small portion of rice or pasta.
   - **Protein**: Aids in muscle support. Examples: Greek yogurt, eggs, lean meats, or a protein shake.
   - **Fats**: Keep moderate; too much fat might slow digestion and make you feel sluggish if eaten too close to exercise.
3. **Examples**:
   - Whole grain toast with peanut butter and a banana.
   - A small bowl of oatmeal topped with berries and a splash of milk.
   - Greek yogurt with sliced fruit and a drizzle of honey.
4. **Hydration**: Drink water to ensure you are not starting your workout dehydrated.

11.6 During-Workout Nutrition

Most moderate workouts under an hour do not require eating mid-exercise. However, if you are exercising longer (like a 90-minute run or bike ride) or doing very intense intervals, you may need extra carbs to maintain energy:

- **Sports Drinks or Water**: Water is enough for shorter sessions. A sports drink with electrolytes and carbs can help in longer or more intense sessions.
- **Easily Digestible Carbs**: Some endurance athletes consume energy gels, chews, or bananas during a race or long event.
- **Listen to Your Body**: If you feel lightheaded or your performance drops, you might need a carb boost.

11.7 Post-Workout Nutrition

Recovery nutrition helps repair muscles, replenish glycogen, and support overall health:

1. **Refuel Within ~30–60 Minutes** (the sooner, the better)
    - This is when muscles are most receptive to replacing glycogen.
2. **Carbs + Protein**
    - A roughly 3:1 or 4:1 ratio of carbs to protein is often suggested for endurance recovery.
    - Strength trainers may focus on 20–30 grams of protein after a workout, along with some carbs.
3. **Examples**:
    - A smoothie with fruit, Greek yogurt or protein powder, and milk (dairy or plant-based).
    - Chicken (or tofu) with brown rice and vegetables.
    - Tuna sandwich on whole grain bread with sliced tomato.
4. **Longer Recovery for Intense Exercise**

- If you completed a marathon or a very intense event, you may need to keep adding carb-rich meals or snacks for the next 24–48 hours to fully replenish glycogen.

11.8 The Importance of Hydration

Water carries nutrients, helps regulate body temperature, and removes waste. Even a small level of dehydration (like 1–2% of body weight) can reduce performance:

1. **General Guidelines**:
   - Drink water regularly throughout the day, not just when you feel thirsty.
   - A rough guideline is about 2.7 liters of total fluids per day for women, but needs vary by climate, activity level, and personal factors.
2. **Exercise and Sweat Rate**:
   - If you sweat heavily or exercise in hot conditions, you need more fluids and possibly electrolytes (like sodium and potassium).
   - Weigh yourself before and after a workout to see if you lost water weight. Drink enough to replace that loss.
3. **Sports Drinks**:
   - Helpful for high-intensity or long workouts, providing electrolytes and a small amount of carbs.
   - For everyday exercise under an hour, water is usually fine.

11.9 Special Considerations for Women Athletes

Women athletes, whether recreational or competitive, should be aware of unique factors:

1. **Menstrual Cycle and Performance**:

- Some women feel more energized during certain phases of their cycle, while others struggle with fatigue or cramps.
- Track your cycle to see patterns. You might adjust workout intensity or rest days accordingly.
- Adequate iron is crucial, especially if you have heavy periods.

2. **Female Athlete Triad / RED-S (Relative Energy Deficiency in Sport):**
    - Occurs when energy intake is too low compared to energy output, leading to menstrual irregularities, low bone density, and possible injuries.
    - Signs include missed periods, fatigue, frequent injuries, and disordered eating patterns.
    - Prevent this by eating enough calories, especially if you are training hard. Focus on carbs and protein, and monitor your cycle.
3. **Pregnancy and Postpartum:**
    - Moderate exercise is often recommended during pregnancy (with doctor approval), but energy needs go up slightly.
    - Postpartum exercise can help with recovery, but the body needs proper nutrition—especially if breastfeeding.

11.10 Balancing Exercise and Rest

Exercise is beneficial, but rest and recovery are equally important:

1. **Overtraining Syndrome**
    - Symptoms: Persistent fatigue, irritability, trouble sleeping, weaker performance.
    - Can lead to injuries or hormonal imbalances if you never let your body recover.
2. **Active Recovery**

- Light activities (gentle yoga, stretching, walking) can help circulation without overloading muscles.
3. **Quality Sleep**
    - Aim for 7–8 hours of sleep. Muscle repair, hormone regulation, and mental recovery all occur during rest.
4. **Nutrition During Rest Days**
    - Keep fueling with balanced meals. You might lower total calories slightly if you are less active, but do not skip meals or severely cut back if your overall schedule is consistent.

11.11 Signs of Underfueling or Poor Nutrition

- **Chronic Fatigue**: Feeling tired even after adequate rest could indicate not enough calories or imbalanced nutrients.
- **Frequent Illness**: A weak immune system might be linked to insufficient vitamins, minerals, or overall calories.
- **Menstrual Irregularities**: Missed or irregular periods may signal a chronic energy deficit.
- **Injuries**: Stress fractures and overuse injuries can occur if bones and muscles are not supported with proper nutrients.
- **Mood Swings**: Low energy intake might affect mood and concentration.

If you recognize these signs, consider talking to a health professional or a registered dietitian to review your eating habits and exercise schedule.

11.12 Building Sustainable Exercise Habits

1. **Start Small**
    - If you are new to exercise, begin with 2–3 short sessions per week. Gradually increase time or intensity.
2. **Find Activities You Enjoy**

- Variety keeps you engaged—maybe dancing, hiking, swimming, or group classes. If you hate running, try something else.
3. **Set Clear Goals**
    - Maybe you want to run a 5K, do 10 push-ups, or attend a yoga class twice a week. Having goals keeps you motivated.
4. **Track Progress**
    - Keep a workout log or use an app to see improvements over time—this can be very motivating.
5. **Stay Flexible**
    - Life happens; if you miss a workout, do not beat yourself up. Adjust and continue.

CHAPTER 12: EMOTIONAL EATING AND BODY IMAGE

12.1 Understanding Emotional Eating

Many women turn to food for comfort during times of stress, sadness, boredom, or even happiness. This is called **emotional eating**—using food to cope with or enhance emotions rather than to satisfy actual physical hunger. Emotional eating in itself is not "bad," but it can become problematic if it leads to overeating, guilt, or a cycle of unhealthy behaviors.

In this chapter, we will explore what triggers emotional eating, the difference between physical and emotional hunger, and strategies to develop a healthier relationship with food. We will also discuss body image—how you see and feel about your body—and ways to cultivate a positive self-view that supports overall well-being rather than undermines it.

12.2 Physical Hunger vs. Emotional Hunger

Physical hunger grows gradually. You might feel your stomach rumble or experience a dip in energy. Emotional hunger, on the other hand, can appear suddenly, often paired with an intense craving (like needing chocolate right away).

- **Physical Hunger**:
    1. Builds slowly.
    2. Open to various foods.
    3. Stops when you are full.
    4. Leaves no guilt afterward.
- **Emotional Hunger**:
    1. Hits suddenly.

2. Usually linked to specific "comfort foods" (often high in sugar, fat, or salt).
3. Persists even after you are physically full.
4. Might lead to guilt or shame afterward.

Recognizing which type of hunger you feel is the first step toward mindful eating.

12.3 Common Triggers for Emotional Eating

1. **Stress**: When stress hormones like cortisol are elevated, cravings for high-energy foods can intensify.
2. **Boredom**: Eating can become a way to fill time or break monotony.
3. **Sadness or Loneliness**: Food might temporarily distract from feelings of emptiness or low mood.
4. **Celebrations and Social Events**: Sometimes emotional eating is positive—like indulging at a party—but it can lead to overconsumption.
5. **Habits and Associations**: If you always ate ice cream after a tough day in childhood, you might continue that pattern as an adult.

12.4 Body Image: What It Is and Why It Matters

Body image refers to how you see your physical self—whether you feel confident, ashamed, or somewhere in between. It can be influenced by society, media, friends, and family. A **positive body image** means accepting your body and appreciating what it does, rather than being overly fixated on perceived flaws.

12.4.1 Why Body Image Is Important

- **Mental Health**: A negative body image can lead to low self-esteem, anxiety, or depression.

- **Physical Health**: If you dislike your body, you might avoid exercise or try extreme diets, which can harm health.
- **Social Life**: Poor body image may make you withdraw from social activities or avoid certain events.

12.4.2 Influences on Body Image

- **Media and Social Media**: Unrealistic images or filters can push you to compare yourself to an edited ideal.
- **Family and Friends**: Comments (even jokes) about weight or appearance can shape how you see yourself.
- **Personal Experiences**: Bullying, medical issues, or past trauma can color your self-perception.

12.5 The Emotional Eating Cycle

Understanding the cycle can help you break it:

1. **Trigger/Emotion**: You feel stressed, bored, or sad.
2. **Craving**: You believe a certain food (like chocolate or chips) will help you feel better.
3. **Action**: You eat the food—sometimes quickly, without paying attention to hunger cues.
4. **Temporary Relief**: You get a brief sense of comfort or distraction.
5. **Regret/Guilt**: You might feel bad about what or how much you ate.
6. **New Emotions**: Guilt or shame can become triggers, repeating the cycle.

12.6 Strategies to Cope with Emotional Eating

1. **Identify Triggers**
   - Keep a journal to note what happened and how you felt before you had an urge to eat. Look for patterns.
2. **Find Alternatives**

- Instead of eating, try going for a short walk, doing a quick breathing exercise, calling a friend, or writing in a journal.
3. **Delay**
    - Wait 10–15 minutes before grabbing a snack. Sometimes the craving passes or weakens.
4. **Mindful Eating**
    - If you choose to eat, do it slowly. Savor each bite. This can reduce the likelihood of overeating.
5. **Plan Healthy Comfort Foods**
    - If you know you often crave sweets under stress, keep fruit or a small portion of dark chocolate on hand instead of a large container of ice cream.
6. **Seek Support**
    - Talking to a therapist, joining a support group, or confiding in a friend can help process emotions instead of burying them under food.

12.7 Cultivating a Positive Body Image

1. **Shift Your Focus**
    - Instead of obsessing about what you dislike, think about what your body can do. Can you walk, dance, hug loved ones, or create art? These are wonderful abilities.
2. **Challenge Negative Thoughts**
    - If you catch yourself thinking, "I hate my thighs," ask yourself if that thought is fair or true. Could you replace it with something kinder, like, "My legs let me stand, walk, and move through the day"?
3. **Surround Yourself with Positivity**
    - Fill your social media feeds with body-positive accounts. Avoid or unfollow pages that make you feel worse about yourself.
4. **Compliment Yourself**

- This might feel strange at first, but saying or writing down positive affirmations about yourself can build self-esteem over time.
5. **Wear Clothes That Fit Comfortably**
    - Clothes that pinch or feel too tight can constantly remind you of body anxieties. Properly fitting outfits can help you feel more at ease.

12.8 Mindful Eating Techniques

Mindful eating helps you stay in the present moment:

1. **Slow Down**
    - Put your fork down between bites. Chew thoroughly. Pay attention to the texture and taste of each bite.
2. **Eliminate Distractions**
    - Turn off the TV and silence your phone. Focus on the act of eating.
3. **Check In With Yourself**
    - Mid-meal, pause and ask: "Am I still hungry? Am I enjoying this?"
4. **Respect Fullness**
    - Stop eating when you feel satisfied, not stuffed.
5. **Practice Gratitude**
    - Appreciate the food on your plate—where it came from, how it was prepared, and how it nourishes your body.

12.9 Handling Cravings in a Healthy Way

Cravings can be tricky. Sometimes they arise from boredom, stress, or habit rather than true hunger.

1. **Opt for Healthier Versions**
    - If you crave something sweet, try fresh berries, a small piece of dark chocolate, or yogurt with honey.

2. **Use the "5-Minute Rule"**
   - Wait 5 minutes to see if the craving passes. During that time, drink water or do a short task.
3. **Portion Control**
   - If you really want ice cream, serve a small bowl instead of eating straight from the container.
4. **Balance the Meal**
   - Sometimes cravings are stronger if your previous meal was unbalanced or too small. Ensure each meal has protein, complex carbs, and healthy fats to keep you satisfied.

12.10 When Professional Help May Be Needed

If emotional eating is severe, leading to frequent binge episodes or significant distress, or if poor body image affects your daily life, professional intervention may be wise:

- **Therapists/Counselors**: Can offer cognitive-behavioral therapy (CBT), dialectical behavior therapy (DBT), or other approaches to address the root emotions and coping mechanisms.
- **Registered Dietitians**: Can guide you on balanced meal plans and mindful eating practices.
- **Support Groups**: Community-based groups (in person or online) where people share experiences and strategies for dealing with similar issues.

12.11 Steps to Improve Body Image

1. **Challenge Cultural Norms**
   - Realize that beauty standards change over time and differ by culture. There is no single "ideal" shape or size.
2. **Limit Comparison**

- Comparing yourself to others (especially on social media) can fuel negative self-talk. Learn to admire others without putting yourself down.

3. **Practice Self-Care**
    - Activities like taking a bath, reading a book, gentle stretching, or creative hobbies can help you appreciate your body's abilities rather than criticize its appearance.
4. **Focus on Health, Not Perfection**
    - Set goals like "I want to feel more energetic and move more easily," rather than aiming for a specific clothing size or a number on the scale.

12.12 Real-Life Examples of Emotional Eating and Body Image Journeys

Example 1: The Busy Mom

- **Scenario**: A mother of two who rarely gets time for herself. She feels stressed with work, kids, and household responsibilities.
- **Emotional Eating Trigger**: After putting the kids to bed, she feels the day's stress and reaches for cookies or chips.
- **Strategies**:
    - She starts a journal to identify her stress triggers (often after tough days at work).
    - Instead of snacking, she tries a 10-minute bedtime yoga routine or calls a friend for support.
    - She prepares healthier snack options like cut-up fruit or whole grain crackers with cheese.
- **Result**: Over time, she notices that her cravings after the kids' bedtime diminish. She still enjoys occasional treats but is more mindful about them.

Example 2: The College Student

- **Scenario**: A student dealing with exams, social life pressures, and living away from family for the first time.
- **Body Image Concern**: She frequently compares herself to social media influencers and feels inadequate. She also notices she eats late-night fast food when studying.
- **Strategies**:
    - She unfollows certain social media accounts that make her feel bad about her body.
    - She creates a more balanced schedule, including short study breaks for stretching or taking a walk.
    - She sets up a small "study snack kit" with nuts, fresh fruits, and water to replace high-calorie fast foods.
- **Result**: Her late-night binges become less frequent, and she feels more confident. She still uses social media but follows accounts that promote body diversity and mental health.

Example 3: The Young Professional

- **Scenario**: A woman in her late 20s, starting her career. She eats out frequently with colleagues and has a demanding workload.
- **Emotional Eating Trigger**: After a stressful day at work, she orders a large pizza or grabs pastries from a local bakery.
- **Strategies**:
    - She decides to try meal prepping once a week so she has healthy meals ready at home.
    - She practices mindful eating by slowing down and paying attention to flavors, especially during lunch with coworkers.
    - She addresses her stress at work by talking with a mentor and setting boundaries for her workload.
- **Result**: She notices less impulsive eating, saves money, and has more energy during the day. Her sense of body image also improves as she feels more in control.

12.13 Dealing with Setbacks

Improving emotional eating habits and body image is not a straight path. Setbacks happen:

- **Avoid All-Or-Nothing Thinking**: If you have a day of stress eating, do not label yourself a failure. One meal or day does not define your overall progress.
- **Reflect, Don't Dwell**: Consider what led to the setback (lack of sleep, extra stress). Make a plan for next time.
- **Celebrate Small Wins**: Did you manage a craving differently today? Did you notice a kinder thought about your body? Those are victories.

12.14 Building a Supportive Environment

1. **Communicate Your Goals**
    - Tell friends or family about your efforts to reduce emotional eating or improve body image. They might help you find healthier ways to handle stress or celebrate achievements.
2. **Positive Relationships**
    - Spend more time with people who uplift you, not those who constantly criticize your weight or looks.
3. **Organize Your Space**
    - If possible, keep junk food out of easy reach. Stock your fridge with healthy, convenient options.
4. **Consider Professional Guidance**
    - A counselor or dietitian can help personalize strategies and keep you motivated.

12.15 Reframing Exercise and Food

Sometimes, negative body image or emotional eating comes from seeing food and exercise as punishment or reward:

- **Food is Nourishment**
    - Instead of thinking "I have to burn off these calories," see food as fuel and exercise as a way to feel strong and energetic.
- **Exercise is Self-Care**
    - Rather than "I must go to the gym to fix my body," think "I move my body because it boosts my mood and keeps me healthy."

12.16 Overcoming Cultural and Social Pressure

Many cultures celebrate thinness or certain body shapes as the ideal. This can be harmful if it leads to shame or extreme dieting:

1. **Recognize Diverse Body Types**
    - People come in all shapes and sizes. Health is not limited to one body form.
2. **Speak Up**
    - If family or friends make harmful comments about weight, respectfully share how it affects you. Request that they refrain from body-shaming talk.
3. **Educate Yourself**
    - Learn about "Health at Every Size" (HAES) or body neutrality movements that focus on overall well-being instead of just weight.

12.17 Mindset Shifts and Self-Compassion

1. **Be Kind to Yourself**
    - Treat yourself like you would a dear friend. You would offer support, not harsh criticism, if a friend felt bad about her body.
2. **Avoid Perfectionism**
    - Striving to be perfect in diet or appearance can lead to burnout. Aim for progress, not perfection.
3. **Acknowledge Your Feelings**

- Instead of pushing away sadness or stress, admit it. If you feel lonely, let yourself feel it, then look for a healthy response.
4. **Practice Gratitude**
    - Each day, list a few things you appreciate about your body or your life—maybe your resilience, strong arms, ability to laugh, or a good conversation.

12.18 Balancing Healthy Eating with Enjoyment

A healthy relationship with food means allowing for occasional treats without guilt:

1. **Honor Cravings Occasionally**
    - If you truly crave ice cream, have a single serving. Being too restrictive can backfire, leading to binges.
2. **Enjoy Social Outings**
    - Food is part of culture and bonding. You can attend parties or dinners and still respect your body. Try to include fruits and veggies alongside the fun foods.
3. **Moderation vs. Deprivation**
    - Total deprivation of favorite foods can increase obsession. Moderate portions fit into a balanced lifestyle.

CHAPTER 13: ADDRESSING COMMON NUTRITIONAL DEFICIENCIES

13.1 Introduction to Nutritional Deficiencies

Nutritional deficiencies happen when the body does not receive enough of a certain nutrient. Even when you think you are eating a balanced diet, daily life factors—stress, busy schedules, hormonal fluctuations—can lead to gaps. In this chapter, we will discuss common deficiencies that affect women, the symptoms they cause, and practical steps to correct or prevent them.

Because a woman's body undergoes various changes over a lifetime—menstruation, pregnancy, menopause—the risk of certain deficiencies can be higher. For example, women of childbearing age might be more prone to iron deficiency due to monthly blood loss. Pregnant women need extra folate and iron for the baby's development. Postmenopausal women need to keep a close eye on calcium and vitamin D for bone health. Being aware of these possible nutrient gaps empowers you to make informed choices about your diet and supplementation if needed.

13.2 Iron Deficiency

Iron is vital for making hemoglobin, a protein that helps red blood cells carry oxygen around the body. Women of reproductive age often lose iron through menstrual bleeding, which can lead to or worsen iron deficiency. Pregnant women also need extra iron for fetal growth.

13.2.1 Signs and Symptoms

- **Fatigue and Weakness**: Feeling tired after normal activities or having trouble concentrating.
- **Pale Skin**: Especially noticeable in the face, the lining of the eyes, or nail beds.
- **Brittle Nails**: Nails that break easily or look thinner.
- **Shortness of Breath**: You might feel winded doing tasks that you previously handled well.
- **Frequent Headaches**: Caused by reduced oxygen supply to the brain.

13.2.2 Food Sources

- **Heme Iron**: Found in animal products like red meat, poultry, and fish. This type of iron is more easily absorbed.
- **Non-Heme Iron**: Found in beans, lentils, spinach, fortified cereals, tofu, and nuts. Absorption can be boosted by pairing with **vitamin C** (e.g., tomatoes, citrus fruits).

13.2.3 Prevention and Correction

- **Varied Meals**: Include both animal and plant sources of iron if possible. If you follow a vegetarian or vegan diet, make sure to pair iron-rich foods with vitamin C-rich foods.
- **Supplements**: If blood tests confirm low iron, a healthcare provider might recommend an iron supplement. High doses can cause stomach upset or constipation, so follow medical advice.
- **Cooking Methods**: Using cast-iron cookware can slightly increase the iron content of foods.

13.3 Vitamin D Deficiency

Vitamin D helps the body absorb calcium, supports bone health, and may play a role in immune function. Women can be at risk of vitamin

D deficiency if they do not get enough sunlight exposure or if their diet lacks vitamin D–fortified foods or fatty fish.

13.3.1 Signs and Symptoms

- **Bone or Muscle Pain**: Achiness, especially in the lower back, hips, or legs.
- **Frequent Illnesses**: Possible lowered immunity.
- **Fatigue and Low Mood**: Some research links low vitamin D levels with feeling tired or "down."
- **Bone Density Loss**: Long-term deficiency can contribute to osteoporosis, especially in postmenopausal women.

13.3.2 Sources of Vitamin D

- **Sunlight**: The skin produces vitamin D when exposed to UVB rays. About 10–15 minutes of midday sun on arms and legs a few times a week can help, but this varies by location, skin tone, and sunscreen use.
- **Foods**: Fatty fish (salmon, sardines, mackerel), egg yolks, mushrooms exposed to UV light, and fortified products (milk, orange juice, cereals).
- **Supplements**: Vitamin D3 is often recommended if blood levels are low, especially during winter or for those who get limited sun.

13.3.3 Prevention and Correction

- **Safe Sun Exposure**: Brief, moderate exposure is helpful, but sun protection is also important to prevent skin damage.
- **Dietary Choices**: Include vitamin D–rich and fortified foods regularly.
- **Testing**: A simple blood test can measure vitamin D levels. If you are deficient, your doctor might advise a supplement or a higher dose for a short period.

13.4 Calcium Deficiency

Calcium is crucial for bone health, muscle function, and nerve signaling. Women risk developing weak bones (osteoporosis) if their long-term calcium intake is too low, particularly after menopause.

13.4.1 Signs and Symptoms

- **No Early Clear Symptoms**: Calcium deficiency can be silent until bone density gets very low.
- **Possible Muscle Cramps**: In some people, low calcium may show up as muscle spasms or cramps.
- **Bone Fractures**: Over time, weaker bones can increase the chance of fractures.
- **Brittle Nails**: Nails may break easily if calcium is consistently low.

13.4.2 Food Sources

- **Dairy**: Milk, cheese, and yogurt.
- **Fortified Plant Milks**: Soy, almond, oat, or rice milk often have added calcium.
- **Leafy Greens**: Kale, collard greens, bok choy.
- **Sardines and Canned Salmon**: Bones in canned fish are soft and edible, providing a calcium boost.

13.4.3 Prevention and Correction

- **Aim for Consistent Intake**: Spread calcium-rich foods throughout the day to maximize absorption.
- **Pair with Vitamin D**: Without enough vitamin D, calcium absorption can suffer.
- **Weight-Bearing Exercise**: Activities like walking, jogging, or light weightlifting stress bones in a good way, helping maintain density.
- **Supplements**: A calcium supplement may be advised if dietary intake is insufficient. However, excessive calcium

supplementation can raise the risk of kidney stones, so follow medical guidance.

13.5 Vitamin B12 Deficiency

Vitamin B12 supports nerve function, red blood cell formation, and DNA production. Women following plant-based diets, older adults, or anyone with certain digestive conditions may be more likely to have B12 deficiency.

13.5.1 Signs and Symptoms

- **Fatigue and Weakness**: Similar to iron deficiency anemia.
- **Numbness or Tingling**: Hands and feet may feel pins and needles, reflecting nerve issues.
- **Memory Problems**: Severe deficiency might affect thinking or memory.
- **Pale or Jaundiced Skin**: The complexion might look pale, or mild jaundice can appear in some cases.

13.5.2 Food Sources

- **Animal Products**: Meat, fish, poultry, eggs, dairy.
- **Fortified Foods**: Some cereals, nutritional yeast, or plant milks contain added B12.

13.5.3 Prevention and Correction

- **Regular Intake**: If you are vegetarian or vegan, rely on fortified foods or supplements.
- **Blood Tests**: B12 levels can be measured. If they are low, your doctor may suggest oral supplements or even injections in severe cases.
- **Watch for Absorption Issues**: Conditions like pernicious anemia or certain gastrointestinal problems can affect B12 absorption.

13.6 Magnesium Deficiency

Magnesium contributes to many body processes, including muscle relaxation, nerve function, energy production, and bone structure. Stress, a diet high in processed foods, or certain medical conditions can lower magnesium levels.

13.6.1 Signs and Symptoms

- **Muscle Cramps or Spasms**: Especially in the legs, feet, or hands.
- **Fatigue and Weakness**: Low magnesium may also affect energy.
- **Mood Changes**: Some research links inadequate magnesium with anxiety or irritability.
- **Abnormal Heart Rhythms**: In severe cases, low magnesium can alter heart function.

13.6.2 Food Sources

- **Leafy Greens**: Spinach, Swiss chard, kale.
- **Nuts and Seeds**: Almonds, pumpkin seeds, sunflower seeds.
- **Legumes**: Beans and lentils.
- **Whole Grains**: Brown rice, oats, whole wheat bread.

13.6.3 Prevention and Correction

- **Whole Foods First**: A diet rich in vegetables, grains, nuts, and seeds often covers magnesium needs.
- **Check Calcium Intake**: Excessive calcium or certain medications can lower magnesium.
- **Supplement Carefully**: Some forms of magnesium supplements can cause diarrhea if taken in large amounts, so follow recommended doses.

13.7 Folate (Vitamin B9) Deficiency

Folate is essential for cell growth, DNA production, and preventing certain birth defects in pregnant women. Women of childbearing age are often advised to keep folate intake high in case of pregnancy.

13.7.1 Signs and Symptoms

- **Fatigue and Anemia**: Similar to B12 and iron deficiency.
- **Weakness**: Low folate can reduce red blood cell production.
- **Mouth Sores**: Some people get painful sores inside the mouth or a swollen tongue.

13.7.2 Food Sources

- **Leafy Greens**: Spinach, romaine lettuce, collard greens.
- **Legumes**: Lentils, chickpeas, black beans.
- **Fortified Grains**: Many cereals, breads, or flours have added folic acid.
- **Citrus Fruits**: Oranges, grapefruits.

13.7.3 Prevention and Correction

- **Eat a Variety of Plant Foods**: Include legumes and leafy greens in meals.
- **Prenatal Vitamins**: Women planning a pregnancy or who could become pregnant often take a supplement containing folic acid.
- **Avoid Overcooking**: Prolonged heat can reduce folate content in foods. Light steaming or quick sautéing helps preserve nutrients.

13.8 Omega-3 Fatty Acid Deficiency

Omega-3 fatty acids (like EPA and DHA) support heart and brain health, reduce inflammation, and may help with mood regulation.

Women may be low in omega-3s if they rarely eat fish or other sources.

13.8.1 Signs and Symptoms

- **Dry Skin and Hair**: Could include flaky scalp or brittle hair.
- **Mood Changes**: Some research suggests low omega-3 intake might correlate with higher rates of depression or anxiety.
- **Joint Pain**: Omega-3s help reduce inflammation.
- **Poor Concentration**: Cognitive function could be affected.

13.8.2 Sources

- **Fatty Fish**: Salmon, mackerel, sardines, trout.
- **Plant Sources**: Flaxseeds, chia seeds, walnuts, hemp seeds (these mostly provide ALA, which the body converts to EPA and DHA at lower efficiency).
- **Algae-Based Supplements**: A direct source of DHA and EPA for vegans.

13.8.3 Prevention and Correction

- **Regular Fish Intake**: Aim for two servings of fatty fish per week, if you eat fish.
- **Plant Options**: Use ground flaxseeds or chia seeds in smoothies or oatmeal.
- **Consider a Supplement**: Fish oil or algae-based omega-3 supplements can help if diet alone is insufficient.

13.9 Recognizing Overlaps and Multiple Deficiencies

It is possible to be deficient in more than one nutrient at a time. For example, a woman might have low iron, low vitamin D, and low magnesium simultaneously. This can happen with restrictive diets, chronic stress, digestive problems, or certain medications.

Key points if you suspect multiple deficiencies:

- Get blood work done to pinpoint what is truly low.
- Consult a healthcare provider or a registered dietitian for a tailored plan.
- Gradually introduce or increase foods high in needed nutrients.
- Use supplements if recommended, but be careful of potential interactions (for instance, too much calcium can hinder iron absorption if taken at the same time).

13.10 Lifestyle Factors Affecting Deficiencies

1. **Stress**: Chronic stress can deplete certain nutrients like magnesium or B vitamins.
2. **Lack of Sleep**: Poor sleep quality might worsen metabolic issues and reduce nutrient absorption or appetite control.
3. **Smoking or Excessive Alcohol**: Can interfere with absorption of vitamins and minerals or increase the body's nutrient requirements.
4. **Digestive Disorders**: Conditions like Crohn's disease or celiac disease might impair nutrient uptake.

13.11 Testing and Diagnosing Deficiencies

If you suspect a deficiency, a blood test is often the best way to confirm. Examples include:

- **Complete Blood Count (CBC)**: Checks for anemia, which can signal iron or folate issues.
- **Ferritin Test**: Measures iron stores.
- **Vitamin D (25-OH) Test**: Shows vitamin D status.
- **Vitamin B12 Test**: Evaluates B12 levels.
- **Calcium and Magnesium Levels**: Measured through routine blood tests, though results might not always reflect total body stores accurately.

- **Thyroid Function**: Not a vitamin or mineral test per se, but thyroid imbalances can affect overall nutrition.

13.12 Practical Steps to Avoid Deficiencies

1. **Eat a Variety of Whole Foods**: Aim for different colors of fruits and vegetables, whole grains, lean proteins, and healthy fats.
2. **Avoid Extreme Restrictive Diets**: Cutting out entire food groups can boost the risk of deficiencies. If you do avoid certain groups (like dairy), plan alternatives.
3. **Mindful Cooking**: Overcooking can destroy vitamins, especially water-soluble ones like vitamin C and some B vitamins. Use gentler cooking methods when possible.
4. **Pair Nutrients Wisely**: For example, vitamin C boosts iron absorption, and vitamin D helps calcium uptake. On the other hand, calcium and iron taken together can interfere with each other's absorption. Space out those supplements if needed.
5. **Consider Fortified Foods**: Cereals, breads, and plant milks fortified with vitamins and minerals can fill in gaps.
6. **Supplements as a Safety Net**: If recommended by your doctor, use supplements carefully. More is not always better; some vitamins and minerals can be harmful in excess.

13.13 Real-Life Example

A Busy Working Woman

- **Lifestyle**: She grabs quick meals at her office cafeteria, rarely sees the sun because she goes to work early and leaves late, and often feels tired. She recently noticed hair thinning and was told her iron levels are borderline low.
- **Actions**:
    1. She visited her doctor, who confirmed iron deficiency anemia and low vitamin D.

2. She added more iron-rich foods (like lentils and spinach) to her lunch, pairing them with an orange to boost iron absorption.
3. She started a short midday walk outside for 10–15 minutes of sunlight.
4. After follow-ups, her doctor prescribed a low-dose iron supplement and recommended vitamin D supplementation.
- **Outcome**: Within a few months, her energy improved, hair thinning lessened, and blood tests showed her nutrient levels moved closer to normal ranges.

13.14 Over-Supplementation: A Word of Caution

While undernutrition is a concern, taking too many supplements can also harm health:

- **Vitamin A Toxicity**: Can lead to vision issues, headaches, or even liver damage if extremely high.
- **Vitamin D Excess**: High doses over time may cause calcium buildup in the blood, leading to confusion, heart rhythm problems, or kidney damage.
- **Iron Overload**: Can damage organs, especially in people with certain genetic conditions (like hemochromatosis).

Always follow recommended guidelines and consult with a healthcare professional if unsure.

CHAPTER 14: PREGNANCY AND POSTPARTUM NUTRITION

14.1 Why Nutrition Is Crucial During Pregnancy and Postpartum

Pregnancy marks a remarkable change in a woman's body. You are growing another human being, and that requires extra nutrients, careful attention to what you eat, and possibly some lifestyle adjustments. During the postpartum period, your body works to recover from childbirth and, if you choose to breastfeed, to produce milk that nourishes the baby. This chapter explores how to meet these demands by focusing on balanced meals, key nutrients, and practical tips for busy new mothers.

Many women think of pregnancy nutrition as just "eating more," but quality matters more than quantity. You do not need to double your calories—rather, you need to ensure that the calories you do eat are nutrient-dense. Later, in postpartum, your body transitions again, and the demands shift. Hormones fluctuate, sleep is often disrupted, and your schedule might be packed with newborn care. Knowing how to plan meals and address common challenges (like fatigue or low appetite) can support a smoother journey.

14.2 Pre-Pregnancy and Early Pregnancy Considerations

1. **Folate (Folic Acid)**
    - **Importance**: Helps prevent neural tube defects (like spina bifida).
    - **Recommendation**: Women who may become pregnant often take 400–600 micrograms of folic acid daily, starting before conception.
2. **Balanced Diet**

    - **Why**: A healthy body at conception sets the stage for better fetal development. Aim for varied whole foods, lean proteins, whole grains, fruits, and vegetables.
 3. **Healthy Weight**
    - **Reason**: Being significantly underweight or overweight can impact ovulation and increase risks during pregnancy.
 4. **Medical Check-Ups**
    - **Action**: A doctor may run blood tests to check iron levels, thyroid function, and other factors. This is a good time to address any deficiencies (like low vitamin D or B12).

14.3 Key Nutrients During Pregnancy

14.3.1 Protein

- **Role**: Builds and repairs tissues, supports fetal growth (including the placenta).
- **Sources**: Lean meats, fish, poultry, eggs, beans, lentils, dairy products, and tofu.
- **Recommended Intake**: In the second and third trimesters, protein needs increase. Aim for about 70 grams daily (this can vary based on body size).

14.3.2 Iron

- **Role**: Red blood cells carry oxygen to the baby.
- **Sources**: Lean red meat, beans, fortified cereals, spinach.
- **Considerations**: Pair with vitamin C-rich foods to boost absorption. Iron supplements might be necessary if blood work shows anemia.

14.3.3 Calcium

- **Role**: Fetal bone and tooth development, as well as the mother's bone health.

- **Sources**: Dairy, fortified plant milks, leafy greens, sardines.
- **Recommended Intake**: Around 1,000 mg a day for most adults; pregnant teens may need more.

14.3.4 Vitamin D

- **Role**: Helps the body use calcium effectively, supports bone health, and may have immune benefits.
- **Sources**: Fortified milk, fatty fish, sunlight exposure. Supplements might be necessary in areas with low sunlight or for those with confirmed deficiency.

14.3.5 DHA (an Omega-3 Fat)

- **Role**: Fetal brain and eye development.
- **Sources**: Fatty fish (salmon, sardines), fish oil or algae-based supplements.
- **Note**: Some fish can be high in mercury (like shark, swordfish). Choose lower-mercury options.

14.3.6 Folate

- **Role**: Cell division and growth. Prevents neural tube defects.
- **Sources**: Leafy greens, legumes, fortified cereals.
- **Supplementation**: Often recommended in a prenatal vitamin.

14.4 Foods to Limit or Avoid

1. **High-Mercury Fish**: Swordfish, king mackerel, tilefish, shark. Mercury can harm the baby's developing nervous system.
2. **Unpasteurized Dairy and Soft Cheeses**: Risk of listeria, which can cause serious infections.
3. **Raw or Undercooked Meats**: Risk of bacteria and parasites (like toxoplasma).
4. **Excess Caffeine**: Some guidelines suggest limiting to about 200 mg of caffeine per day (about one 12-ounce cup of coffee).

5. **Alcohol**: No safe level has been established during pregnancy; complete avoidance is advised to prevent fetal alcohol syndrome.

14.5 Managing Common Pregnancy Issues with Nutrition

1. **Morning Sickness**
   - *Tip*: Small, frequent meals. Bland, starchy foods like crackers may help. Ginger tea can relieve nausea for some.
2. **Heartburn**
   - *Tip*: Avoid spicy or acidic foods if they trigger symptoms. Eat smaller meals. Do not lie down immediately after eating.
3. **Constipation**
   - *Tip*: Increase fiber (fruits, vegetables, whole grains) and water intake. Gentle exercise can also help.
4. **Cravings or Aversions**
   - *Tip*: If cravings are not harmful, moderate indulgence is usually fine. For nutrient-poor cravings (like very sugary foods), try healthier alternatives or portion control.
5. **Fatigue**
   - *Tip*: Balanced meals and snacks, staying hydrated, and checking for iron deficiency if exhaustion is severe.

14.6 Weight Gain Recommendations During Pregnancy

Overall weight gain varies by pre-pregnancy BMI and health status. Doctors often provide personalized guidelines, but general ranges might be:

- **Underweight (BMI <18.5)**: Aim for 28–40 pounds (about 13–18 kg).

- **Normal Weight (BMI 18.5–24.9)**: Aim for 25–35 pounds (about 11–16 kg).
- **Overweight (BMI 25–29.9)**: Aim for 15–25 pounds (about 7–11 kg).
- **Obese (BMI ≥30)**: Aim for 11–20 pounds (about 5–9 kg).

Gaining too little can risk low-birth-weight babies; too much can lead to complications like gestational diabetes or hypertension. Focus on nutrient-rich foods rather than empty calories.

14.7 Nutrition and Gestational Diabetes

Gestational diabetes occurs when the body cannot handle blood sugar effectively during pregnancy. It typically appears in the second or third trimester. Nutrition plays a major role:

- **Control Carbohydrates**: Emphasize complex carbs (whole grains, beans, vegetables) over refined sugary foods.
- **Balance Meals**: Pair carbs with protein or healthy fats to slow glucose spikes.
- **Monitor Blood Sugar**: Working closely with a healthcare provider or dietitian helps manage levels to keep mom and baby healthy.
- **Exercise**: Light to moderate activities, with medical approval, can improve insulin sensitivity.

14.8 Postpartum Nutrition and Recovery

After birth, the body is healing from pregnancy and labor. Hormones fluctuate, and if breastfeeding, you are using extra energy to produce milk.

1. **Increased Caloric Needs** (if breastfeeding)
   - Producing breast milk can burn an additional 300–500 calories per day. But focus on quality, not just quantity.

2. **Protein and Nutrient Density**
   - Helps tissue repair and supports energy. Lean meats, beans, eggs, and dairy or dairy alternatives can be central.
3. **Hydration**
   - Breastfeeding requires more fluids. Keep a water bottle handy.
4. **Balanced Snacks**
   - Newborns feed often, so convenient snacks (like cut-up fruits, nuts, whole grain crackers, cheese) help meet constant hunger in a healthy way.

14.9 Breastfeeding: Important Nutrients and Considerations

1. **Calcium**
   - The body may draw from the mother's bones if intake is insufficient, risking bone density loss. Aim for adequate calcium plus vitamin D.
2. **Iron**
   - Menstruation may not return immediately while breastfeeding, but iron stores might still be low after pregnancy. Monitor iron levels.
3. **Vitamin B12**
   - Crucial if you are vegan or vegetarian, since B12 is mainly from animal foods or fortified products. Low maternal B12 can affect the baby's growth and development.
4. **Omega-3s (DHA)**
   - Support baby's brain development through breast milk.
5. **Caffeine and Alcohol**
   - Small amounts may pass into breast milk. Experts often suggest limiting caffeine to a moderate amount and avoiding alcohol or timing it carefully after a feed.

14.10 Addressing Postpartum Challenges

1. **Postpartum Fatigue**
   - Interrupted sleep combined with recovery from childbirth can cause extreme tiredness. Nutrient-rich snacks and possibly iron checks are important.
2. **Mood Changes**
   - The "baby blues" or postpartum depression can occur. While nutrition alone cannot fix severe depression, stable blood sugar and essential nutrients (like omega-3s) may support better mood. Seek professional help if symptoms worsen.
3. **Weight Loss Pressure**
   - Society often pushes new moms to "bounce back." However, postpartum recovery takes time. Gentle exercise, balanced eating, and patience are more sustainable than drastic measures.
4. **Limited Time for Meal Prep**
   - Newborn care is all-consuming. Consider batch cooking, asking friends or family for help with meals, or keeping healthy frozen options on hand.

14.11 Special Diets During Pregnancy and Postpartum

- **Vegetarian/Vegan**: Must pay extra attention to iron, B12, calcium, and omega-3s. Use fortified foods and possibly supplements.
- **Gluten-Free**: For celiac or gluten sensitivity, ensure you get enough nutrients from other grains (like quinoa, brown rice) plus fruits, vegetables, and proteins.
- **Lactose Intolerance**: Choose calcium-fortified plant milks or lactose-free dairy products to meet calcium and vitamin D needs.

- **Low-Carb or Keto**: Typically not recommended during pregnancy unless medically supervised. Can lack essential nutrients for fetal development.

14.12 Real-Life Example

A First-Time Mom's Journey

- **Situation**: She starts pregnancy slightly overweight. She struggles with morning sickness in the first trimester but craves sweets in the second.
- **Actions**:
    - Works with a dietitian to incorporate more protein and complex carbs.
    - Takes a prenatal vitamin with folic acid, iron, and DHA.
    - When sweet cravings strike, she opts for fruit first or small servings of dark chocolate.
    - Exercises gently (walking, prenatal yoga) with her doctor's okay.
- **Postpartum**:
    - She breastfeeds, noticing she feels extra hungry. She keeps trail mix and protein bars in a nursing station. She also cooks in batches (soups, stews) to save time.
    - Her postpartum check-ups show stable iron levels. While she has not lost all baby weight immediately, she focuses on eating well and caring for her newborn.

14.13 Meal Planning Tips for Pregnancy and Postpartum

1. **Small, Frequent Meals**: Especially helpful during pregnancy if heartburn or nausea is an issue. Post-birth, frequent meals or snacks align with a busy infant care schedule.
2. **Include a Protein Source at Each Meal**: Helps stabilize blood sugar and supports tissue repair. Examples: eggs for breakfast, chicken or beans for lunch, fish or tofu for dinner.

3. **Snack Smart**: Think of nutrient-dense options—yogurt with fruit, whole grain crackers with cheese, hummus with veggies, or nuts and seeds.
4. **Use Time-Savers**: Frozen vegetables, canned beans, or pre-chopped produce can simplify cooking.
5. **Stay Hydrated**: Water, flavored seltzers, herbal teas, and broth-based soups can help meet fluid needs.

14.14 Emotional Well-Being and Support

- **Ask for Help**: Let partners, family, or friends know you need meal assistance or grocery runs.
- **Seek Professional Care**: If mood swings, depression, or severe anxiety occur, talk to a doctor or counselor. Nutrition is only part of the puzzle.
- **Online and Local Groups**: Breastfeeding or new-mom groups often share meal ideas and coping strategies.
- **Celebrate Small Wins**: Maybe you tried a new healthy recipe or found a 15-minute window for a walk. These small steps add up.

14.15 Returning to Exercise Postpartum

- **Doctor's Clearance**: Typically 6 weeks after normal delivery, longer if there were complications or a C-section.
- **Gentle Start**: Walks, pelvic floor exercises, and light stretching are good beginnings.
- **Fuel Your Body**: Post-workout snacks or meals with carbs and protein support recovery, especially while breastfeeding.
- **Avoid Rapid Weight Loss Goals**: Remember that your body is still healing; focus on gradual progress.

14.16 When to Consult a Professional

- **Ongoing Digestive Issues**: Prolonged morning sickness or hyperemesis gravidarum requires medical attention.

- **Significant Weight Fluctuations**: Sudden weight gain or loss might indicate an underlying issue (gestational diabetes, preeclampsia, postpartum thyroid problems).
- **Nutrient Deficiencies**: If blood tests show low iron, vitamin D, or any other essential nutrient, a dietitian can craft a personalized plan.
- **Breastfeeding Challenges**: A lactation consultant can help if you struggle with low milk supply or breastfeeding pain, which might reduce your appetite or fluid intake.

14.17 Cultural Foods and Preferences

Pregnancy and postpartum traditions vary worldwide. If you have cultural favorites:

- **Adapt Recipes**: Substitute healthier cooking methods (baking instead of frying) or lower-sodium ingredients where possible.
- **Keep the Nutrient Core**: Many traditional postpartum foods are rich in herbs, spices, and warming ingredients that can offer comfort and potentially aid digestion. Just balance them with other nutrient-rich staples.
- **Ask Elders**: Family recipes or remedies may offer soothing properties. Combine cultural wisdom with modern nutritional guidelines to strike a healthy balance.

14.18 Addressing Myths

1. **"You're Eating for Two"**: This does not mean doubling your calories. In reality, caloric needs only moderately increase—by about 300 extra calories a day in the second trimester and a bit more in the third, depending on your situation.
2. **"Cravings Must Be Obeyed"**: Cravings can signal some nutrient needs, but often they are just comfort desires. Moderation is key.

3. **"No Exercise Allowed"**: Most healthy pregnancies benefit from light to moderate exercise, but always consult with a medical professional.
4. **"Breastfeeding Guarantees Weight Loss"**: While it does burn extra calories, hormonal shifts and personal factors mean postpartum weight loss varies widely.

14.19 Long-Term Perspective

Pregnancy and the postpartum period are relatively short in the span of a lifetime, yet they greatly impact health. Setting good habits now can help:

- **Model Healthy Behaviors**: If you continue these habits as your child grows, you teach them by example.
- **Future Pregnancies**: If you choose to have more children, knowledge gained here carries over.
- **Overall Well-Being**: Balanced nutrition and self-care support not only the baby but also your mental and physical health.

CHAPTER 15: MENOPAUSE AND BEYOND

15.1 Understanding Menopause and Its Stages

Menopause is a natural transition in a woman's life when her ovaries gradually reduce hormone production, particularly estrogen and progesterone. It typically occurs in a woman's late 40s or early 50s, though timing can vary. Menopause is officially defined as the point in time when a woman has gone 12 consecutive months without a menstrual period. The process leading up to this point is **perimenopause**, and the phase after is often called **postmenopause**.

Perimenopause can last for several years. During this time, hormone levels fluctuate, and you may experience irregular periods, hot flashes, night sweats, mood swings, and other symptoms. Once you reach menopause—no periods for 12 months—your body settles into a low-estrogen state called postmenopause. Some symptoms (like hot flashes) may become less frequent over time, but others (like decreased bone density) might show up more clearly in the long run.

Menopause is not a disease but a normal part of aging. Yet the drop in estrogen can increase certain health risks, such as decreased bone density and higher chances of cardiovascular problems. Nutrition, exercise, and lifestyle adjustments can help manage symptoms and maintain health during and after this transition.

15.2 Key Nutritional Concerns During Menopause

1. **Bone Health**
    - **Why It Matters**: Estrogen has a protective effect on bones. As levels fall, women risk accelerated bone loss, which can lead to osteopenia or osteoporosis.

- **How to Support**: Adequate calcium, vitamin D, magnesium, and weight-bearing exercises are vital. Foods like milk, leafy greens, and fortified plant milks help, but you may also need supplements if diet alone is insufficient.

2. **Cardiovascular Health**
   - **Why It Matters**: Estrogen also helps maintain healthy cholesterol levels and blood vessel function. After menopause, risks for heart disease may increase.
   - **How to Support**: Focus on whole grains, lean proteins, fruits, vegetables, nuts, seeds, and healthy fats (like olive oil). Limit saturated and trans fats, and stay active to keep blood pressure and cholesterol in check.

3. **Weight Management**
   - **Why It Matters**: Hormone changes can make it easier to gain weight around the abdomen. Metabolism may slow, and muscle mass often declines with age.
   - **How to Support**: Balanced meals with sufficient protein, coupled with regular exercise—especially strength training—helps preserve muscle and manage weight.

4. **Hot Flashes and Night Sweats**
   - **Why It Matters**: Fluctuations in hormone levels can trigger sudden waves of heat and sweating.
   - **How to Support**: Some women find relief by avoiding triggers like spicy foods, caffeine, or alcohol. Staying hydrated and dressing in layers can help manage symptoms.

5. **Mood and Energy**
   - **Why It Matters**: Hormonal shifts can affect mood, stress levels, and energy.
   - **How to Support**: Steady blood sugar (by eating balanced meals), regular exercise, and nutrients like B

vitamins, omega-3 fats, and magnesium may help stabilize mood and reduce fatigue.

15.3 The Role of Specific Nutrients in Menopause

1. **Calcium**
   - **Function**: Maintains bone structure.
   - **Food Sources**: Dairy, fortified milks, tofu made with calcium sulfate, leafy greens, canned fish with soft bones (sardines, salmon).
   - **Daily Target**: Around 1,200 mg for postmenopausal women (though this can vary). Divide intake between meals for better absorption.
2. **Vitamin D**
   - **Function**: Helps the body absorb calcium, supports the immune system, and may influence mood.
   - **Food Sources**: Fatty fish (salmon, mackerel), fortified products, egg yolks.
   - **Sun Exposure**: Skin makes vitamin D when exposed to sunlight, but factors like age, location, sunscreen use, and skin tone affect production.
   - **Supplementation**: Many postmenopausal women take vitamin D3 if blood levels are low.
3. **Protein**
   - **Function**: Maintains muscle mass, which is crucial as muscle may decline with age. Also supports bone health by interacting with hormones that protect bones.
   - **Food Sources**: Lean meats, fish, eggs, dairy, legumes, soy products, nuts, seeds.
   - **Amount**: Some experts suggest aiming for 1–1.2 grams of protein per kilogram of body weight daily as you age, but needs vary.
4. **Phytoestrogens**

- **Function**: Plant compounds that mimic mild estrogen in the body. They may help some women ease mild hot flashes or other symptoms, though results differ.
- **Food Sources**: Soy (tofu, tempeh, edamame), flaxseeds, legumes.
- **Caution**: Phytoestrogens are not as potent as human estrogen. Talk to a healthcare provider if you have a history of estrogen-sensitive conditions.

5. **B Vitamins**
    - **Function**: Energy metabolism, nerve function, and possibly mood support.
    - **Food Sources**: Whole grains, legumes, nuts, seeds, lean meats, fortified cereals.
    - **Note**: Folic acid (B9) and B12 are especially important to support healthy blood cells and nerve function in older age.

15.4 Managing Symptoms Through Diet and Lifestyle

1. **Hot Flashes**
    - **Triggers**: Caffeine, spicy foods, alcohol, or very hot beverages might exacerbate flashes.
    - **Cooling Foods**: Hydration is key. Fresh fruits, vegetables, and herbal teas can support fluid balance.
    - **Lifestyle**: Dressing in layers, using a fan, or practicing controlled breathing when a hot flash hits can bring relief.
2. **Night Sweats and Sleep Disruption**
    - **Tips**: Avoid heavy meals or caffeine close to bedtime. Keep the bedroom cool and well-ventilated.
    - **Calming Teas**: Chamomile or lavender tea might help relaxation, though they do not necessarily reduce night sweats directly.
    - **Mind-Body Practices**: Light yoga or meditation before bed may improve sleep quality.

3. **Mood Swings and Emotional Well-Being**
   - **Nutritional Support**: Ensure steady intake of complex carbs, protein, and healthy fats to keep blood sugar stable.
   - **Physical Activity**: Regular exercise releases endorphins that can boost mood and help manage stress.
   - **Social Connections**: Menopause can be emotionally challenging. Finding supportive friends, family, or counselors helps reduce feelings of isolation.
4. **Midlife Weight Gain**
   - **Approach**: Rather than extreme diets, focus on nutrient-dense foods, portion control, and routine physical activity (like brisk walking or water aerobics).
   - **Muscle Preservation**: Strength training two or three times a week helps counter muscle loss and supports metabolism.
   - **Mindful Eating**: Pay attention to hunger and fullness cues. Emotional eating might intensify during menopause, so addressing stress with non-food strategies (journaling, gentle exercise, talking with a friend) can help.

15.5 Specific Life Changes After Menopause

1. **Bone Density Tests**
   - **When**: Doctors might recommend a bone density scan (DEXA) to assess osteoporosis risk.
   - **Why**: Early detection of bone loss can guide interventions, like boosting calcium and vitamin D or discussing medications with a doctor.
2. **Heart Health Monitoring**
   - **Blood Pressure Checks**: Make sure to monitor regularly. High blood pressure can sneak up with age.

- **Cholesterol Levels**: Keep an eye on LDL ("bad") cholesterol, HDL ("good") cholesterol, and triglycerides. Nutritional changes and physical activity can help manage these.
3. **Hormone Replacement Therapy (HRT)**
    - **Overview**: Some women consider HRT to ease severe symptoms. However, it has risks and benefits, so it is a personal decision made with a healthcare provider.
    - **Nutrition and HRT**: Even with therapy, good nutrition remains crucial to support overall health.
4. **Joint Health**
    - **Concern**: Age-related joint stiffness or pain can coincide with menopause.
    - **Nutrients**: Omega-3 fats (from fish or supplements), plus fruits and veggies with antioxidants, may help reduce inflammation.
    - **Gentle Exercise**: Activities like swimming or yoga can ease joint stiffness.

15.6 Mental and Emotional Shifts

Menopause can bring changes in self-image and confidence, especially in a culture that often celebrates youth. Recognizing this natural transition and adjusting health habits can foster a sense of control and well-being.

- **Body Image**: Appreciating your body for its strengths (like carrying you through decades of life) rather than focusing on aging changes can improve self-esteem.
- **Stress Management**: Meditation, deep breathing, or creative hobbies can release tension and support better hormonal balance.
- **Seeking Support**: Menopause support groups or talking with a counselor can help if mood swings or anxiety feel overwhelming.

15.7 Sample Menopause-Friendly Meals

Below is an example day that focuses on key nutrients for menopausal and postmenopausal women:

1. **Breakfast**:
    - Whole grain oatmeal topped with ground flaxseeds (phytoestrogens and omega-3s), a handful of blueberries (antioxidants), and a drizzle of almond butter (healthy fats).
    - A side of low-fat or plant-based yogurt fortified with calcium and vitamin D.
2. **Snack**:
    - Apple slices with a tablespoon of peanut butter (protein, healthy fats).
    - Herbal tea, like chamomile or mint.
3. **Lunch**:
    - Spinach salad with grilled salmon (calcium in spinach, omega-3s and vitamin D in salmon), sliced strawberries, walnuts (healthy fats, omega-3), and a light vinaigrette dressing.
    - Whole grain crackers or a small whole wheat roll on the side.
4. **Snack**:
    - Low-fat cheese stick (calcium, protein) and carrot sticks (fiber, vitamins).
    - Water with cucumber slices.
5. **Dinner**:
    - Stir-fry made with tofu (phytoestrogens), bell peppers, broccoli, onions, and a light garlic-ginger sauce. Serve over brown rice.
    - A side of steamed edamame (extra protein, more phytoestrogens).
6. **Optional Dessert**:
    - A small square of dark chocolate or fresh fruit bowl.

- Decaf green tea, which provides antioxidants without the caffeine that might disrupt sleep.

15.8 Physical Activity Recommendations

- **Aerobic Exercise**: Aim for at least 150 minutes per week of moderate-intensity activities (brisk walking, dancing, cycling). This supports heart health and helps manage weight.
- **Strength Training**: At least 2 sessions a week, focusing on major muscle groups to maintain muscle mass and bone strength.
- **Flexibility and Balance**: Yoga, Pilates, or simple stretching routines can improve joint mobility, balance, and overall well-being, reducing the risk of falls.

15.9 Common Myths About Menopause

1. **"Weight Gain Is Unavoidable"**
   - Fact: While it may be easier to gain weight, healthy eating and regular exercise can significantly reduce unwanted weight gain.
2. **"Soy Foods Will Solve All Your Menopause Problems"**
   - Fact: Soy can offer mild relief for some women, but it is not a guaranteed cure. Results vary, and it is only one piece of an overall approach.
3. **"Menopause Symptoms End Immediately After You Stop Having Periods"**
   - Fact: Some women experience hot flashes and other symptoms for years after their last period.
4. **"Calcium Supplements Alone Will Protect Your Bones"**
   - Fact: Vitamin D, magnesium, exercise, and an overall balanced diet are also vital for bone health.

CHAPTER 16: BOOSTING IMMUNITY THROUGH FOOD

16.1 Why Immune Health Matters for Women

A strong immune system helps protect you from viruses, bacteria, and other pathogens. It also plays a role in repairing tissues and managing inflammation. Women face unique immune challenges—menstruation, pregnancy, breastfeeding, and hormonal shifts across life stages can all affect how the immune system functions. Stress, busy schedules, and even certain lifestyle habits (like poor sleep) can weaken immunity over time.

This chapter explores how nutrition impacts the immune system, pointing out specific vitamins, minerals, and other dietary factors known to support your body's defenses. We will also look at lifestyle practices (like adequate sleep and stress reduction) that, along with a nutrient-rich diet, can help you stay healthier throughout the year.

16.2 Basics of the Immune System

1. **Innate Immunity**
    - **Definition**: Your body's first line of defense, which includes physical barriers (like skin) and specialized cells that attack invaders quickly.
    - **Influence of Nutrition**: Nutrient deficiencies can weaken these barriers; for instance, low vitamin A may impair skin health, while low protein may reduce production of immune cells.
2. **Adaptive Immunity**
    - **Definition**: Involves antibodies and specialized cells (like T-cells) that remember specific pathogens and mount stronger attacks with each exposure.

- **Influence of Nutrition**: Vitamins and minerals (like vitamins C and D, zinc, and others) support the growth and function of these immune cells, helping the body respond effectively.

3. **Inflammation**
    - **Role**: A controlled inflammation response helps the body fight infection or heal injuries.
    - **Issue**: Chronic or excessive inflammation can damage tissues. Diets high in added sugars, refined carbs, or unhealthy fats can contribute to chronic inflammation, while antioxidant-rich diets can help reduce it.

16.3 Nutrients That Support Immune Function

1. **Vitamin C**
    - **Role**: Known for boosting white blood cell production, reducing oxidative stress, and supporting skin barriers.
    - **Sources**: Citrus fruits, bell peppers, broccoli, strawberries, kiwi.
    - **Practical Tips**: Vitamin C is water-soluble, so daily intake is important since the body does not store large amounts.
2. **Vitamin D**
    - **Role**: Helps activate immune cells and regulate inflammation. Low levels have been linked with increased susceptibility to infections.
    - **Sources**: Fatty fish, fortified foods, egg yolks, sunlight exposure.
    - **Caution**: If you live in a region with limited sunlight, or you have darker skin, supplementation might be necessary. A blood test can confirm deficiency.

3. **Zinc**
    - **Role**: Critical for the development and function of immune cells like T-cells. Also involved in wound healing.
    - **Sources**: Oysters, lean red meat, pumpkin seeds, chickpeas, fortified cereals.
    - **Note**: Excessive zinc supplementation can interfere with copper absorption, so stay within recommended limits unless directed by a doctor.
4. **Vitamin A**
    - **Role**: Maintains mucous membranes (in the eyes, respiratory tract, gut), which are important barriers against infections.
    - **Sources**: Orange and yellow fruits/vegetables (carrots, sweet potatoes, mangoes), dark leafy greens, eggs, fortified dairy.
    - **Safety**: Too much preformed vitamin A (like from certain supplements) can be toxic. Beta-carotene from plants is safer because the body converts it to vitamin A as needed.
5. **Vitamin E**
    - **Role**: Antioxidant that helps protect cells from damage, supports healthy blood vessels, and may improve certain immune functions.
    - **Sources**: Nuts, seeds (sunflower seeds, almonds), vegetable oils, spinach, avocados.
    - **Recommendation**: Aim to get vitamin E from foods rather than high-dose supplements to avoid imbalances.
6. **Selenium**
    - **Role**: Supports antioxidant enzymes that fight oxidative stress and can enhance immune response.
    - **Sources**: Brazil nuts (they are very high in selenium), seafood, poultry, whole grains, sunflower seeds.

- **Warning**: Because Brazil nuts are extremely high in selenium, it is easy to exceed the daily limit if you eat them in large amounts regularly.
7. **B Vitamins**
    - **Role**: Involved in energy production, cell growth, and the creation of antibodies. For example, B6 (pyridoxine) supports over 100 enzyme reactions, many related to immunity.
    - **Sources**: Whole grains, poultry, fish, legumes, eggs, dark leafy greens.
8. **Protein**
    - **Role**: Needed to build immune cells and antibodies.
    - **Sources**: Lean meats, fish, beans, lentils, soy products, dairy.
    - **Practical Approach**: Include some protein at each meal or snack to maintain muscle mass and immune cell production.

16.4 Other Immune-Boosting Factors in Foods

1. **Antioxidants**
    - **Why**: They protect cells from damage by free radicals. A broad range of antioxidants can be found in colorful fruits and vegetables (berries, beets, bell peppers).
    - **Categories**: Flavonoids, polyphenols, carotenoids, and more—each type offers different protective benefits.
2. **Probiotics**
    - **Function**: Beneficial bacteria that support gut health. A large portion of your immune system is in the gut, so a balanced microbiome aids in defense.
    - **Sources**: Yogurt with live cultures, kefir, kombucha, sauerkraut, kimchi, and other fermented foods.
    - **Suggestion**: Consuming probiotic-rich foods regularly might improve gut barrier function, but more research is ongoing.

3. **Prebiotics**
   - **Function**: Indigestible fibers that feed the beneficial bacteria in your gut.
   - **Sources**: Onions, garlic, leeks, asparagus, bananas, whole grains.
   - **Why**: Supporting gut bacteria with prebiotics indirectly bolsters immune health, as a healthy microbiome can reduce inflammation and help guard against pathogens.
4. **Omega-3 Fatty Acids**
   - **Role**: Anti-inflammatory properties can help regulate immune responses. Chronic inflammation can hinder immunity, so balancing omega-3 and omega-6 fats is important.
   - **Sources**: Salmon, mackerel, sardines, flaxseeds, chia seeds, walnuts, algae-based supplements.

16.5 Foods and Habits That Weaken Immunity

1. **Excess Sugar**
   - **Issue**: Spikes in blood sugar may temporarily reduce white blood cell efficiency. Over the long term, high-sugar diets contribute to inflammation and obesity, both of which can compromise immunity.
   - **Tip**: Limit sugary drinks, desserts, and excessive use of sweeteners.
2. **Processed Foods**
   - **Issue**: High in refined flours, unhealthy fats, additives, and low in essential nutrients. They can promote inflammation and fail to provide the vitamins and minerals your body needs.
   - **Tip**: Opt for whole foods like fruits, vegetables, whole grains, and lean proteins whenever possible.

3. **Excess Alcohol**
   - **Issue**: Alcohol can disrupt gut bacteria, impair nutrient absorption, and reduce white blood cell production if consumed heavily.
   - **Tip**: Moderation is key. Some guidelines recommend no more than one drink per day for women, but even less is preferable for optimal immune function.
4. **Trans Fats and Excessive Saturated Fats**
   - **Issue**: Linked to heart disease risk and inflammation, potentially weakening overall immunity.
   - **Tip**: Check labels for "partially hydrogenated oils" and choose healthier oils (olive, avocado) and nuts/seeds instead of fried or processed fatty foods.

16.6 Lifestyle Factors Affecting Immunity

1. **Sleep**
   - **Why**: During sleep, your body produces and releases cytokines (proteins that help fight infection and inflammation). Lack of sleep can reduce the production of these protective proteins.
   - **Goal**: Aim for 7–8 hours of quality sleep. If you have trouble sleeping, consider reducing caffeine later in the day and practicing a calming bedtime routine.
2. **Stress Management**
   - **Why**: Chronic stress triggers cortisol release, which can lower immune function over time.
   - **How**: Techniques like deep breathing, meditation, exercise, journaling, or spending time in nature can reduce stress hormones and support a stronger immune system.
3. **Physical Activity**
   - **Benefit**: Moderate exercise increases circulation of immune cells, helping them patrol the body more effectively. It also reduces inflammation.

- **Balance**: Excessive intense exercise might temporarily weaken immunity, so aim for moderation—about 150 minutes of moderate activity or 75 minutes of vigorous activity per week, plus strength training.
4. **Healthy Weight**
    - **Reason**: Obesity can lead to chronic low-grade inflammation, weakening immune defenses.
    - **Approach**: Combine nutrient-dense eating with regular physical activity to maintain or reach a healthy body composition.
5. **Clean Environment**
    - **Tip**: Wash hands regularly, keep kitchen surfaces sanitized, and properly handle food to prevent infections that can overload or confuse the immune system.

16.7 Building a Daily Immune-Supportive Meal Plan

Below is a sample one-day plan focusing on immune-boosting nutrients:

1. **Breakfast**:
    - Oatmeal with sliced strawberries (vitamin C), sunflower seeds (vitamin E, selenium), and a drizzle of honey.
    - Low-fat yogurt or a small glass of kefir for probiotics.
2. **Mid-Morning Snack**:
    - An orange or kiwi for extra vitamin C.
    - A handful of walnuts (omega-3 fats and protein).
3. **Lunch**:
    - Lentil and vegetable soup (lentils for protein and iron, carrots and tomatoes for vitamin A and antioxidants).
    - Side of whole grain bread or crackers.
    - A small spinach salad with bell peppers (vitamin C) and a drizzle of olive oil dressing.
4. **Afternoon Snack**:

- Apple slices with almond butter (vitamin E, protein, healthy fats).
- Green tea for its catechins (antioxidants).

5. **Dinner**:
    - Baked salmon (rich in omega-3s) with a lemon-garlic sauce.
    - Steamed broccoli (vitamin C, fiber) topped with a little olive oil.
    - Quinoa or brown rice on the side (B vitamins, protein).
6. **Evening Wind-Down**:
    - Chamomile tea (may promote relaxation and better sleep).
    - Small square of dark chocolate (antioxidants) if desired, in moderation.

16.8 Immune-Supportive Herbs and Spices

1. **Garlic**
    - **Active Compounds**: Allicin and other sulfur-containing substances believed to have antimicrobial and immune-modulating effects.
    - **Use**: Fresh crushed garlic in dressings, stir-fries, or soups. Cooking reduces some potency, but it still offers flavor and some benefits.
2. **Ginger**
    - **Properties**: Anti-inflammatory, may help soothe digestive upsets.
    - **Use**: Grate fresh ginger into teas, soups, or marinades.
3. **Turmeric**
    - **Key Component**: Curcumin, which has anti-inflammatory properties.
    - **Tip**: Combining turmeric with black pepper enhances curcumin absorption. Use it in curries, soups, or golden milk.
4.

5. **Cinnamon**
   - **Potential Effects**: May help regulate blood sugar, and stable blood sugar indirectly supports a balanced immune system.
   - **Use**: Sprinkled on oatmeal, yogurt, or in teas.
6. **Oregano**
   - **Potential Benefits**: Contains antioxidants and may help fight bacteria.
   - **Use**: Fresh or dried in sauces, soups, or roasted vegetables.

16.9 Special Immune Considerations for Women

1. **Pregnancy**
   - The immune system adapts to protect both mother and fetus. Nutrient demands are higher for vitamins and minerals. Focus on iron, folate, and overall balanced meals.
   - Certain herbs or supplements might not be safe during pregnancy—always consult a healthcare provider.
2. **Postpartum**
   - Physical recovery plus the demands of caring for a newborn can stress immunity. Adequate protein, vitamins, and minerals support healing. Hydration is crucial, especially when breastfeeding.
3. **Perimenopause and Menopause**
   - Hormonal changes can affect inflammation and bone health. High-antioxidant diets with plenty of calcium, vitamin D, and phytonutrients help reduce inflammatory stress.
4. **Older Women**
   - The immune system weakens with age (immunosenescence). Absorption of nutrients like vitamin B12 may decline. Paying extra attention to

nutrient-dense foods and possibly supplemental support can help maintain immune function.

16.10 Supplements: Are They Necessary?

While a balanced diet is the best way to get nutrients, certain situations may warrant supplements:

- **Confirmed Deficiencies**: A blood test shows low vitamin D, iron, or B12, for example.
- **Restricted Diets**: Vegans may need B12 or iron support. Those with malabsorption issues might need specialized supplements.
- **Busy Lifestyle**: Sometimes a multivitamin can fill small gaps, but it should not replace real food.
- **Illness or Recovery**: Extra vitamin C or zinc might support healing, though it is always wise to consult a healthcare provider.

Caution: Over-supplementation (especially with fat-soluble vitamins A, D, E, and K) can be harmful. Stick to recommended doses.

16.11 Recognizing Immune-Impairing Behaviors

If you find yourself frequently ill, it is worth evaluating:

- **Skipping Meals** or relying on junk food.
- **Chronic Sleep Deprivation** (less than 6 hours most nights).
- **High Stress Levels** with no coping strategies.
- **Excess Alcohol** or smoking.
- **Sedentary Lifestyle** without consistent exercise.

Changing these habits can make a notable difference in how often you get sick and how quickly you recover.

16.12 Role of Hydration in Immune Function

Water transports nutrients to cells and helps remove wastes. Staying hydrated keeps mucous membranes (like those in your respiratory system) moist, providing a better barrier against microbes. Aim for:

- **General Guideline**: Around 2.7 liters of fluid per day for adult women, from water, herbal teas, and water-rich foods (fruits, veggies).
- **Extra Needs**: If you exercise, live in a hot climate, or are pregnant/breastfeeding, you likely require more fluids.

16.13 Stress, Immunity, and Nutrition Connection

Chronic stress raises cortisol levels, which over time can suppress certain immune responses. Nutrient deficiencies further worsen the situation. Strategies for synergy:

- **Balanced Diet**: Stabilizes energy and mood, reducing stress triggers caused by blood sugar swings.
- **Relaxation Techniques**: Try breathing exercises before meals to calm nerves and help digestion.
- **Slow, Mindful Eating**: Enjoying meals without rushing or distractions can reduce stress hormones.

16.14 Myths About Immune-Boosting Foods

1. **"Superfoods" Cure All**
   - Reality: No single food can magically prevent or cure infections. A balanced approach with variety is more effective than relying on one "super" ingredient.
2. **"Massive Vitamin C Doses Prevent Colds Completely"**
   - Reality: While adequate vitamin C supports immunity, mega-doses beyond recommended levels have not definitively proven to stop colds, though they might slightly shorten their duration.

3. **"Only Supplements Can Improve Immunity"**
   - Reality: Supplements may help in some cases, but whole foods, sleep, exercise, and stress management are fundamental.

16.15 Immune Health for Different Life Stages

1. **Adolescence**
   - Rapid growth, menstrual onset. Ensure iron, calcium, and vitamins A and C for strong immune function.
2. **Early to Mid-Adulthood**
   - Busy lifestyles can lead to skipped meals or convenience foods. Balance is key to prevent chronic inflammation and ensure adequate nutrient intake.
3. **Menopause and Beyond**
   - Reduced estrogen can affect inflammatory processes. Antioxidant-rich foods and nutrients that support bone health (calcium, vitamin D) remain critical for overall immune resiliency.

16.16 Putting It All Together: A Holistic Approach

Nutrient-Dense Diet: Fill half your plate with fruits and vegetables, one quarter with protein, and one quarter with whole grains. Rotate different foods to get a full range of nutrients.

Lifestyle Habits: Sleep 7–8 hours, manage stress, avoid smoking, keep alcohol in check, and prioritize regular physical activity to keep immune function strong.

Frequent Handwashing: Though not a diet measure, hygiene is an external factor that complements internal immunity.

16.17 Examples of Immune-Supportive Meal Ideas

1. **Breakfast**: Veggie omelet (spinach, tomatoes, mushrooms) with a side of fresh fruit. This provides protein, vitamins, and antioxidants.
2. **Lunch**: Grain bowl with quinoa, mixed greens, roasted chickpeas (zinc, protein), colorful peppers (vitamin C), a drizzle of tahini (healthy fats, calcium), and a sprinkle of pumpkin seeds (zinc, magnesium).
3. **Snack**: Yogurt parfait layered with berries (antioxidants), a spoonful of honey, and a sprinkle of ground flaxseeds for omega-3s.
4. **Dinner**: Baked chicken breast (lean protein) with a side of sweet potatoes (beta-carotene), sautéed kale (folate, vitamin C), and brown rice (B vitamins).
5. **Dessert**: A small cup of pineapple or papaya for natural enzymes, plus herbal tea.

16.18 Handling Illness and Recovery

If you do catch a cold or the flu:

- **Hydrate**: Warm teas, broths, and water help loosen mucus and prevent dehydration.
- **Gentle Nutrient Intake**: Soups, stews, and smoothies can be easier to eat when appetite is low.
- **Rest**: Quality sleep and reduced stress allow the body to direct energy toward healing.
- **Consult a Professional**: If symptoms worsen or do not improve, see a doctor. Nutrition alone cannot replace medical treatment if a more serious infection or condition is present.

16.19 Addressing Autoimmune Conditions

Women are more likely than men to develop autoimmune disorders (like rheumatoid arthritis, Hashimoto's thyroiditis, or lupus). While each condition is different, certain nutritional approaches may help manage inflammation:

- **Anti-Inflammatory Diets**: Emphasize fruits, vegetables, whole grains, fatty fish, and healthy oils. Avoid foods that trigger inflammation, which can be different for each individual.
- **Food Sensitivities**: Some people with autoimmune conditions find relief by limiting gluten or dairy, but this is highly individual.
- **Professional Guidance**: A registered dietitian familiar with autoimmune disorders can help you identify beneficial foods and avoid potential triggers.

CHAPTER 17: BUILDING HEALTHY HABITS AND SETTING GOALS

17.1 Why Habits Matter for Women's Health

A habit is something you do often and almost automatically. Habits can be helpful, like brushing your teeth every morning, or unhelpful, like grabbing a bag of chips whenever you watch TV. When it comes to nutrition and well-being, forming healthy habits is especially important. It is not just about knowing what to eat but turning that knowledge into regular actions.

For women, daily life can be busy. Some women juggle work, caregiving, studying, or other responsibilities. In these conditions, habits provide a sense of order and allow healthy choices to happen without too much extra thought. If you build a routine around preparing healthy meals, drinking enough water, and being active, you will find it easier to stick to your nutrition goals. Building these habits, however, can take time and patience.

In this chapter, we will explore how to form habits that stick, set goals that motivate you, and keep going when challenges arise. Whether your aim is to eat more vegetables, be more active, or reduce stress, the steps to creating lasting change are similar. By the end, you will have practical ideas to transform small actions into daily habits that bring you closer to better health.

17.2 How Habits Form

Habits come from repeated actions. Each time you do something, your brain forms neural pathways that make the action easier the next time. After enough repetition, you can perform the habit without thinking much about it.

The Habit Loop is commonly described as having three parts:

1. **Cue (Trigger)**: Something that starts the action. For example, getting home from work might cue you to grab a snack.
2. **Routine (Action)**: The behavior you perform in response to the cue (reaching for potato chips or, more helpfully, washing some fresh fruit).
3. **Reward (Benefit)**: The feeling or outcome you get from the action, such as satisfaction or relief from hunger.

Over time, your brain starts to link the cue with the routine and expects the reward. If you want to build a new habit—like drinking more water—setting up a clear cue (for example, always filling a water bottle after breakfast) and recognizing the reward (feeling refreshed) can help. Similarly, to break an unhealthy habit, identify your triggers, replace the routine, and find a healthier reward.

17.3 Setting SMART Goals

Goals give your habits direction. For instance, saying "I want to eat better" is too vague. You are more likely to succeed if you make your goal **SMART**:

1. **Specific**: Clear and detailed. Instead of "eat healthier," say, "eat two servings of vegetables at lunch and dinner each day."
2. **Measurable**: You can track your progress. "Two servings" is measurable; "eat more veggies" is not precise enough.
3. **Achievable**: It should be realistic for your life right now. If you almost never eat vegetables, starting with two servings a day might be more achievable than jumping straight to five.
4. **Relevant**: It should matter to you. If you do not care about vegetables, you might not stay motivated. Pick a goal that supports your personal health priorities.

5. **Time-bound**: Give yourself a timeline. "For the next month, I will have two servings of vegetables at lunch and dinner each day."

When you have a SMART goal, your brain knows exactly what to do and by when. This clarity helps you stay focused. You can also adapt your goal if you find it too easy or too hard. For example, if two servings of veggies at lunch and dinner is too big a leap, try one serving at dinner. Gradually increase as you build confidence.

17.4 Finding Your "Why"

Another part of building habits that stick is knowing your motivation. Some women feel pressured by social media or family members to change their diets or lose weight. But external pressure often does not last. You need to find your own strong reason (your "why") to keep you going. Examples might be:

- **Wanting More Energy**: So you can keep up with your kids or excel at your job.
- **Improving Mood**: So you feel less stressed and more positive day to day.
- **Preventing Future Health Problems**: If high blood pressure or diabetes runs in your family, forming healthy eating patterns can lower your risk.
- **Feeling Strong and Confident**: Maybe you want to build more muscle or simply feel good about your body.

Take a moment to think about why you want to form healthier habits. Write it down or keep it in mind when temptation strikes. Remembering your "why" can push you forward when you would rather give up.

17.5 Starting Small: The Power of Tiny Changes

Change can be overwhelming if you try to overhaul everything at once. Instead, start with small steps—tiny changes you can repeat easily. For instance, if you want to drink more water, begin by having a cup of water first thing in the morning. Once that becomes normal, add another water break mid-morning. Over time, these small behaviors add up.

This method is sometimes called "baby steps" or "tiny habits." Because the steps are so small, you are more likely to do them daily without resistance. And daily repetition is what cements the habit into your routine. Each small success also builds confidence, encouraging you to tackle slightly bigger goals.

17.6 Examples of Small Habit Changes

Below are some ideas of how you can break down bigger changes into small, manageable actions:

1. **Eating More Fruits and Vegetables**
   - Have one fruit with breakfast.
   - Add a side salad to dinner twice a week.
   - Swap chips for carrot sticks or apple slices as a snack once a day.
2. **Increasing Physical Activity**
   - Park farther away from the store to walk extra steps.
   - Take a 10-minute brisk walk after lunch.
   - Do a quick stretch before bed.
3. **Managing Stress**
   - Take three slow, deep breaths when you wake up.
   - Write in a journal for five minutes in the evening.
   - Spend a minute practicing gratitude before dinner.
4. **Drinking More Water**
   - Drink a small glass of water right when you wake up.
   - Keep a refillable water bottle on your desk.

○ Replace one sugary drink per day with water.

Each of these small actions takes little time or effort. Yet doing them regularly can lay the foundation for bigger changes.

17.7 Habit Stacking

"Habit stacking" is a technique where you attach a new habit to an existing one. For example, if you already brush your teeth every morning, you can add a new mini-habit right after brushing your teeth. If you want to do daily squats, decide to do five squats immediately after you put your toothbrush away. The existing habit (teeth brushing) becomes a cue for the new habit (squats).

Some other habit-stacking examples:

- **After You Brew Your Morning Coffee**: Take a moment to stretch or do a short breathing exercise.
- **After You Finish Lunch**: Do a quick 5-minute walk or stand up and move.
- **Before You Start Dinner**: Fill a water glass to sip as you cook.

By linking the new habit to something you already do, you reduce the need to remember or motivate yourself from scratch.

17.8 Tracking Your Progress

Tracking can be a powerful way to see improvement and stay motivated. You can use:

- **A Journal**: Write down each time you complete your new habit.
- **An App**: Many apps help log water intake, meal quality, or exercise. Some send reminders, which can be helpful.
- **A Calendar or Habit Tracker**: Put a checkmark or sticker on days when you successfully follow through.

When you see a row of stickers or checkmarks, it feels rewarding and encourages you not to break the streak. If you miss a day, do not be too hard on yourself—just get back on track the next day.

17.9 Addressing Setbacks

It is normal to slip up or skip a habit sometimes. For example, you might have an overwhelming day at work and forget to pack a healthy lunch. Instead of calling yourself a failure, figure out what went wrong and how to adjust. Perhaps you need to prep lunches in advance or put a reminder on your phone the night before.

The key is to avoid the "all-or-nothing" mindset. Missing one day does not ruin your progress. What matters is getting back to the habit soon. Every day is a fresh start.

17.10 Making Time for Healthy Habits

One common barrier to building habits is feeling you have no time. Yet often, small pockets of time exist in your day that can fit a quick healthy action. Some tips:

1. **Combine Activities**: Listen to a motivational podcast while cooking or walking.
2. **Use Transition Times**: If you commute on public transport, read a healthy recipe or nutrition tips. If you drive, consider audio resources.
3. **Delegate Tasks**: If possible, ask family members to help with certain chores so you free up time for meal prep or a workout.
4. **Simplify Meals**: Cooking at home does not have to be fancy. A quick stir-fry or salad can be nutrient-packed and fast.

17.11 Motivational Techniques

1. **Positive Self-Talk**: Instead of saying, "I can't do this," try, "I'm learning, and each day I'm getting better."
2. **Visual Reminders**: Put a note on your fridge about your goals or hang a visual chart.
3. **Accountability Partners**: Team up with a friend, coworker, or family member who also wants to build healthy habits. Check in with each other on progress.
4. **Reward Yourself**: Choose a non-food reward (like a relaxing bath, new book, or hobby item) after reaching a small milestone.

17.12 Long-Term vs. Short-Term Goals

Many women start with short-term goals (like losing 5 pounds before a wedding), but focusing only on short-term outcomes can lead to yo-yo dieting or frustration. It is also important to set long-term goals that focus on overall health and well-being. Examples:

- **Short-Term**: "Walk 20 minutes a day for the next two weeks."
- **Long-Term**: "Maintain a regular exercise routine to support a healthy heart."

Balance both types of goals: short-term goals keep you motivated, while long-term goals keep you on a steady path toward lasting change.

17.13 Celebrating Small Wins

When you reach a small milestone—like successfully drinking water first thing in the morning for two weeks—celebrate it. The celebration can be as simple as telling yourself, "Great job!" or marking it on a calendar. If it's a bigger achievement (like consistently meal prepping for a month), reward yourself with something you enjoy, such as a relaxing spa day, a new fitness accessory, or a quiet afternoon reading.

Positive reinforcement helps your brain link the new habit with a good feeling, increasing the chance you will keep it up.

17.14 Adjusting Goals as Needed

Life changes, and so can your habits and goals. If you find your current goals are no longer relevant or you have mastered them, adjust upward. If they are too hard, make them more realistic. For example:

- **Original Goal**: "Cook dinner at home five nights a week."
- **If This Is Too Hard**: Reduce to three nights a week, focusing on healthy, simple recipes.
- **If This Is Easy**: Increase to six nights a week or try more challenging recipes for variety.

There is no shame in altering a goal. What matters is that it pushes you enough to grow but not so much that you feel constantly defeated.

17.15 Common Pitfalls and How to Avoid Them

1. **Taking On Too Much at Once**: Trying to overhaul your entire diet and exercise routine overnight can be overwhelming. Start with one or two habits.
2. **All-or-Nothing Thinking**: Believing you have "failed" if you eat one unplanned treat. Remember, consistency over the long term is what counts, not 100% perfection.
3. **Unclear Goals**: Without a measurable target, it is easy to lose direction. Make your goals specific and trackable.
4. **Lack of Support**: Surrounding yourself with people who sabotage your efforts can make it harder. Seek supportive friends or join online communities with similar goals.

5. **Impatience**: Real habit change can take weeks or months. Patience and persistence are key.

17.16 Habit-Building and Emotional Health

Your emotions can strongly affect your habits. Stress, sadness, or boredom might make you want to skip your new routine. Strategies to handle this include:

- **Mindfulness**: Notice how you feel before reaching for junk food. Ask, "Am I actually hungry, or just stressed?"
- **Healthy Stress Outlets**: Instead of emotional eating, try a quick walk, journaling, or talking with a friend.
- **Self-Compassion**: Recognize you are human. If you slip, talk to yourself kindly, and plan for next time.

17.17 Creating a Supportive Environment

Your environment can either make building habits easier or harder. Examples of modifying your environment include:

- **Food Placement**: Keep healthy snacks (like fruit or nuts) at eye level and hide sugary treats in a less convenient spot or not buy them at all.
- **Kitchen Organization**: Place your blender in an easy-to-reach spot if you want to make more smoothies.
- **Workout Clothes Ready**: Lay out exercise clothes or keep them in your car. This small step can remove friction when you decide to work out.
- **Reduce Temptation**: If you do not want to eat chips frequently, do not keep them in the house or buy them only in small single-serving bags.

17.18 Using Technology Wisely

There are many tools and apps that can help you stay on track, such as:

- **Calorie-Tracking Apps**: Record meals, monitor nutrient intake, and note patterns.
- **Step Counters or Fitness Trackers**: Track daily activity or heart rate, prompting you to move more.
- **Reminder Apps**: Set alarms for meal prep, water intake, or bedtime.
- **Online Communities**: Connect with others for recipes, tips, and encouragement.

However, technology can also be overwhelming or lead to perfectionism. If you find yourself anxious about tracking every bite, consider a less detailed approach. Sometimes simple pen-and-paper logs or a basic checklist might feel more relaxed.

17.19 Sustainability: Making Changes That Last

Sustainability means you can see yourself doing the behavior for months or years. Ask these questions:

- **Is My Goal Enjoyable Enough?** If you hate running, do not force it. Try dancing, cycling, or any activity you can enjoy.
- **Can I Fit This Into My Schedule?** If a 60-minute gym routine feels impossible daily, try 20-minute home workouts.
- **Does It Align with My Lifestyle?** Drastic diets often fail because they do not match your social life, family needs, or personal taste.

Building habits you can keep in your daily life for the long run is crucial for lasting health benefits.

CHAPTER 18: OVERCOMING CHALLENGES AND BARRIERS

18.1 Understanding Common Barriers for Women

While building healthy habits sounds straightforward, real-life barriers can stand in the way. Time constraints, money problems, family commitments, or even emotional struggles can pull you off track. For many women, these barriers feel overwhelming. However, once you identify them, you can create strategies to address or work around them. This chapter focuses on practical tips to overcome common challenges and stay on your path to better nutrition and well-being.

All women face some obstacles, but circumstances vary. A single mom may have different hurdles compared to a college student or a woman living in a rural area with limited grocery options. We will look at how to adapt solutions to your unique situation. Even small changes matter: if you cannot control everything, focus on the pieces you can adjust. Over time, each barrier you tackle builds confidence in your ability to handle future challenges.

18.2 Time Constraints

Barrier: Busy schedules with work, family, or school can make it hard to cook meals, exercise, or even plan. Eating fast food or skipping meals might seem like the only options.

Solutions:

1. **Meal Prepping**: Spend one day (or a few hours) each week preparing meals in bulk. Cook a big pot of soup, roast a tray of vegetables, or grill chicken that can be used in different dishes.

2. **Slow Cooker or Instant Pot**: These appliances let you set a meal in the morning and have it ready by evening with minimal effort.
3. **Quick Recipes**: Look for 15- or 20-minute healthy recipes. Stir-fries, salads with protein, or simple pasta dishes can save time.
4. **Utilize Leftovers**: Prepare extra servings at dinner to use for lunch the next day.
5. **Short Workouts**: If you cannot exercise for an hour, do 10–20-minute sessions a few times a day, such as quick walks or online mini-workout videos.

18.3 Financial Constraints

Barrier: Healthy eating is sometimes seen as expensive. Fresh produce, lean meats, or specialty health products can cost more than cheap, processed meals.

Solutions:

1. **Budget-Friendly Foods**: Beans, lentils, eggs, canned tuna, frozen vegetables, and in-season produce are often cheaper yet still nutritious.
2. **Plan Before Shopping**: Make a weekly meal plan and shopping list to avoid impulse buys. Compare unit prices to get the best deals.
3. **Buy in Bulk**: Staples like oats, rice, and beans can be cheaper when purchased in larger quantities. Store them properly so they last.
4. **Limit Waste**: Use up all the ingredients you buy. Freeze extras or turn leftover vegetables into soups or stir-fries.
5. **Discounts and Coupons**: Check local stores or online apps for sales. Sometimes markets reduce prices at the end of the day on fresh items.

18.4 Emotional and Stress-Related Barriers

Barrier: Stress, sadness, or anxiety can lead to emotional eating—reaching for comfort foods or skipping meals. Women with high stress might not have the energy to plan or cook.

Solutions:

1. **Mindful Eating**: Slow down when eating, notice your hunger cues, and consider if you are truly hungry or just stressed.
2. **Stress Reduction Techniques**: Deep breathing, short walks, journaling, or talking to a counselor can help lower stress so it does not sabotage your eating habits.
3. **Alternative Comforts**: If you normally calm anxiety with sugary snacks, replace that habit with a quick cup of tea, a soothing playlist, or a short guided meditation.
4. **Allow Occasional Treats**: Emotional eating might worsen if you ban all "fun" foods. Enjoy a modest portion of your favorite treat once in a while, savoring each bite.

18.5 Social and Cultural Pressures

Barrier: In some families or cultures, food is central to gatherings, celebrations, or traditions. Refusing certain dishes or changing your diet can cause tension or guilt. Peer pressure from friends or coworkers may also push you toward unhealthy choices (for instance, group lunches at fast-food places).

Solutions:

1. **Communicate Your Needs**: Politely let friends or family know you are trying to make healthier choices. Emphasize that you value time with them but want to adapt the food.
2. **Offer to Bring a Dish**: If you are attending a potluck or family dinner, bring a nutritious option you like. This ensures there is something that fits your goals.

3. **Practice Portion Control**: If certain cultural dishes are important to you, have small servings. Focus on vegetables or lean protein to balance the meal.
4. **Suggest Alternatives**: If your friends always pick a fast-food place, propose a different restaurant with healthier options. Or decide to have a light meal before or after the gathering.

18.6 Lack of Support or Sabotage at Home

Barrier: It is hard to maintain healthier habits if household members bring junk food home or scoff at your choices. You might feel alone or undermined if others do not share your goals.

Solutions:

1. **Ask for Understanding**: Talk to your partner, roommate, or family about why these changes matter. Request they respect your plan, even if they do not join it.
2. **Set Boundaries**: If others want certain snacks, have them store them in a separate cabinet or area. Keep your healthy foods front and center.
3. **Lead by Example**: Over time, seeing your improved energy or mood might inspire them to try healthier choices, too.
4. **Find External Support**: If household support is lacking, look for online groups, coworkers, or local communities with similar health goals.

18.7 Limited Access to Healthy Foods

Barrier: Some women live in "food deserts," areas where fresh fruits and vegetables or good grocery stores are not readily available. Transportation or cost can also limit access.

Solutions:

1. **Frozen and Canned Produce**: These can be just as nutritious as fresh (choose low-sodium or no-sugar-added versions). Stock up when available.
2. **Farmers' Markets or Community Gardens**: If possible, check for local markets or community programs that sell produce at discounted rates.
3. **Online Shopping**: If transportation is a challenge, see if you can order groceries online and have them delivered (if available).
4. **Grow Your Own**: Even a small container garden on a windowsill can provide herbs or small vegetables. This is not always feasible for everyone, but can be an option if you have even a bit of space and sunlight.

18.8 Physical Limitations or Health Conditions

Barrier: Some women have injuries, chronic pains, or conditions like arthritis that make cooking, standing for long, or exercising difficult.

Solutions:

1. **Adapted Exercises**: Chair workouts, water aerobics, or gentle stretching can provide movement without stressing joints. A physical therapist can advise safe exercises.
2. **Kitchen Aids**: Tools like jar openers, food processors, or ergonomic utensils can help if you have grip issues or trouble standing.
3. **Meal Delivery Services**: If cooking is too challenging, consider healthy meal deliveries that fit your budget. Alternatively, ask friends or family for help with meal prep.
4. **Focus on What You Can Control**: If you cannot move around easily, pay extra attention to nutrient-rich, portion-controlled meals for weight management or health goals.

18.9 Emotional Barriers: Self-Doubt, Shame, or Comparison

Barrier: Sometimes the biggest obstacle is feeling unworthy or comparing yourself to others. You may feel you lack willpower or get discouraged if you do not see quick results.

Solutions:

1. **Progress, Not Perfection**: Accept that everyone's journey is unique. Celebrate small changes instead of waiting for huge transformations.
2. **Avoid Negative Comparisons**: Unfollow social media accounts that make you feel bad. Seek pages or groups that celebrate diverse body types and realistic health goals.
3. **Self-Compassion Exercises**: Treat yourself like a friend. If a friend made a mistake, you would not judge them harshly; extend the same kindness to yourself.
4. **Seek Professional Support**: A counselor or therapist can help you address deep-seated self-esteem issues or body image struggles.

18.10 Dealing with Plateaus or Slow Progress

Barrier: You might start strong but then hit a plateau, especially if your goal involves weight change or fitness improvements. No visible progress can tempt you to give up.

Solutions:

1. **Reevaluate Your Approach**: Maybe your body adapted. Try changing your workout routine, adding more strength training, or adjusting your calorie intake.
2. **Switch Up Meals**: If you have been eating the same foods, add variety to ensure you get a wide range of nutrients.

3. **Check Habits**: Are you getting enough sleep? Are you sneaking extra snacks?
4. **Focus on Other Measures**: Check how your clothes fit, your energy levels, or your mood improvements. Progress is not always shown on the scale.

18.11 Overcoming "All-or-Nothing" Thinking

Barrier: Feeling that one slip—like a single indulgent meal—ruins everything. This mindset can lead to giving up entirely.

Solutions:

1. **Balanced Perspective**: One unhealthy choice does not undo weeks of good choices. You can pick a healthier option at the next meal.
2. **Practice the 80/20 Rule**: Aim for healthy choices 80% of the time, leaving room for treats or less healthy foods 20% of the time.
3. **Learn from Mistakes**: Instead of shame, use the slip as data. Why did it happen? How can you prevent it next time?

18.12 Involving Family in Overcoming Challenges

If you have a partner, children, or other family members, getting them on board can lighten the burden:

- **Meal Planning Together**: Let them pick some healthy recipes they would enjoy.
- **Shared Grocery Shopping**: Ask older kids or your partner to help pick out fruits and vegetables.
- **Active Outings**: Plan family walks, bike rides, or park visits as weekend fun.
- **Positive Communication**: Explain that these changes are for everyone's well-being and not a punishment.

18.13 Workplace Obstacles

Barrier: Long hours, office snacks, or lunches out can sabotage your nutrition goals. Stress or lack of break time might also reduce your motivation to eat healthy.

Solutions:

1. **Pack Lunch and Snacks**: Preparing your own meals helps control portions and ingredients. Include easy-to-grab options like nuts, yogurt, or chopped vegetables.
2. **Set Reminders**: Every hour, stand up and stretch or drink water. If your job is desk-bound, mini breaks can aid circulation and reduce mindless snacking.
3. **Colleague Support**: Find a coworker with similar goals. You can encourage each other or split tasks like bringing healthy snacks on alternating days.
4. **Use the Facilities**: If your workplace has a microwave or fridge, store healthy frozen meals or leftover dinners.

18.14 Traveling and Dining Out

Barrier: Restaurants, vacations, or business trips often offer limited healthy choices. Portions can be large, and you might feel pressured to indulge with others.

Solutions:

1. **Research Ahead**: Look up menus online before arriving. Choose restaurants with healthier options or plan in advance what you might order.
2. **Portion Control**: Split a meal with someone or ask for a to-go box right away. That way, you only eat half and save the rest for later.
3. **Healthier Options**: Choose grilled, baked, or steamed items over fried ones. Ask for dressings or sauces on the side.

4. **Snack Packing**: On trips, bring nuts, fruit, or whole-grain crackers to avoid relying on junk food at gas stations or airports.

18.15 Maintaining Motivation During Tough Times

Motivation naturally rises and falls. When you feel low or stressed, your healthy habits might slip. Strategies to renew motivation include:

1. **Recall Your "Why"**: Review why you started this journey. Is it for more energy, better health, or setting a good example for loved ones?
2. **Revisit Goals**: If your goals feel stale, refresh them or set a new short-term target.
3. **Celebrate Non-Scale Victories**: Note improved mood, better sleep, or fewer sugar cravings—these wins can be just as important as weight or measurement changes.
4. **Connect with Others**: Talk with a friend who is also making healthy changes. Mutual encouragement can boost morale.

18.16 Handling Special Events and Holidays

Barrier: Holidays and celebrations often revolve around big meals, sugary desserts, and snacks. It can be hard to stick to your plan without feeling left out.

Solutions:

1. **Eat Mindfully**: Take small portions of favorite holiday dishes and savor them slowly.
2. **Bring a Healthy Dish**: At parties, you ensure at least one lighter option is available.
3. **Avoid Skipping Meals**: Starving yourself before a party can lead to overeating later. Instead, have a small, balanced meal so you arrive with stable hunger levels.

4. **Focus on Socializing**: Use gatherings to connect with people rather than focusing solely on the buffet.

18.17 Emotional Support and Professional Help

Sometimes challenges become too large to handle alone:

- **Registered Dietitian or Nutritionist**: A professional can give personalized advice and meal plans.
- **Counselors or Therapists**: If emotional eating or body image issues are deep-rooted, mental health support can be invaluable.
- **Personal Trainers or Fitness Coaches**: If you are unsure how to exercise safely or effectively, a coach can build a custom routine and keep you accountable.

18.18 Technology Aids

We live in an era of many tech solutions:

- **Food Delivery Services**: Some specialize in healthy, pre-portioned meals. This is handy if you lack cooking time or skill.
- **Grocery Delivery**: If you cannot visit the store, consider an app-based service to deliver fresh produce.
- **Workout Apps**: Offer guided exercise routines, from yoga to strength training, often with short sessions that fit busy schedules.

CHAPTER 19: SELF-CARE, MINDSET, AND STRESS MANAGEMENT

19.1 Understanding Self-Care for Women

"Self-care" means paying attention to your own physical, mental, and emotional needs. It is not selfish or lazy. Rather, it allows you to replenish your energy so you can handle life's responsibilities in a healthier way. Women often have multiple roles—whether as professionals, caregivers, partners, or friends—and it can be easy to put their own well-being last. Yet neglecting self-care can lead to burnout, stress, and lowered health over time.

In the context of nutrition and well-being, self-care may include planning healthy meals, setting aside time to exercise, creating mental space to relax, or embracing supportive mindsets that keep you balanced. By treating self-care as a necessary part of life, you can manage stress better, make healthier choices, and maintain the motivation to keep improving. This chapter explores practical self-care strategies, the power of a resilient mindset, and methods to reduce stress for a healthier relationship with food and your body.

19.2 The Link Between Stress, Mindset, and Nutrition

When you experience stress—due to work, family demands, or other pressures—your body releases stress hormones like cortisol. In small doses, this can be helpful. But chronic, long-term stress keeps cortisol high, which can lead to health issues such as:

- **Weakened Immune Function**: Making you more susceptible to illness.

- **Increased Appetite or Cravings**: Many people find themselves craving sweets or fatty foods when cortisol is elevated.
- **Weight Gain**: Particularly around the abdomen, linked to chronic stress.
- **Poor Sleep**: Which further disrupts hormones that regulate hunger and satiety.

Your **mindset** also matters. If you view healthy eating as a chore or punishment, or if you engage in negative self-talk, you might sabotage your efforts. On the other hand, a growth mindset—believing you can learn and improve—can motivate you to keep trying when challenges arise. Self-care practices offer a way to manage stress and develop a more positive outlook, which in turn supports healthier eating patterns and life choices.

19.3 Defining Self-Care: It's Personal

Self-care does not look the same for everyone. Some might picture a spa day, while others find self-care in a solitary walk, journaling, or reading a good book. The important thing is that you choose activities that nourish you. Areas of self-care include:

1. **Physical Self-Care**: Eating balanced meals, being active, getting enough sleep, staying hydrated.
2. **Emotional Self-Care**: Reflecting on your feelings, practicing mindfulness, or talking to a therapist if needed.
3. **Social Self-Care**: Setting boundaries with toxic relationships, spending time with supportive friends, or having alone time if social situations drain you.
4. **Mental/Intellectual Self-Care**: Challenging your brain with new skills, reading, or problem-solving.
5. **Spiritual Self-Care (Optional)**: Engaging in prayer, meditation, or any practice that helps you find meaning and peace.

19.4 Practical Ways to Practice Self-Care Daily

1. **Schedule It**: Put self-care activities on your calendar as you would a doctor's appointment. This signals that it is important and prevents you from ignoring it.
2. **Set Boundaries**: Learn to say no if you truly do not have time or energy for an extra task. Overcommitting can lead to resentment and burnout.
3. **Create Routines**: Morning or evening rituals (like a few minutes of stretching, journaling, or quiet reflection) can ground you.
4. **Micro-Breaks**: Even a few minutes to breathe deeply, look out a window, or stretch can lower stress hormones.
5. **Declutter**: A tidy environment often leads to a clearer mind. Organize your workspace or kitchen to make healthy habits more natural.

19.5 Mindset Shifts for Better Health

Growth Mindset vs. Fixed Mindset

- A **growth mindset** sees abilities as changeable. Challenges become opportunities to learn. If you fail, you believe you can adjust and succeed later.
- A **fixed mindset** believes abilities are static; if you fail, it feels like a permanent flaw. This mindset can cause you to avoid challenges or give up quickly.

To cultivate a growth mindset regarding nutrition and fitness:

- **Embrace Mistakes**: If you skip a workout or indulge in too many sweets, see it as data. Ask: "What triggered that choice, and how can I handle it better next time?"
- **Celebrate Small Wins**: Every healthy meal or short walk is progress.

- **Speak Kindly to Yourself**: Replace "I can't do this" with "I'm learning how to do this" or "I haven't succeeded yet."

19.6 Stress Management Techniques

Life will always have some stress. The goal is not to eliminate stress, but to handle it in healthier ways. Consider these options:

1. **Mindful Breathing**: Close your eyes, inhale for a count of four, hold for four, exhale for four, and hold for four. Repeat several times.
2. **Yoga or Gentle Stretching**: Releases tension in muscles and promotes relaxation.
3. **Progressive Muscle Relaxation**: Tense and then relax each muscle group, from your feet up to your head.
4. **Journaling**: Writing down worries or gratitude can help process emotions.
5. **Nature Walks**: Studies show being outdoors, especially in green spaces, reduces stress hormones.
6. **Music or Arts**: Listening to calming music or engaging in a creative hobby can shift your focus and reduce anxiety.

19.7 Emotional Eating and Stress Relief

When stress hits, many women turn to "comfort foods" high in sugar, fat, or salt. While this might provide temporary relief, it can lead to guilt or health issues long term. To break the cycle:

- **Pause Before Eating**: Ask yourself if you are truly hungry or just stressed.
- **Identify Emotions**: Are you anxious, sad, or bored? Try a non-food strategy first.
- **Find Healthy Comforts**: Herbal tea, a warm bath, or a short relaxation exercise might provide soothing without sabotaging nutrition.

- **Portion Control**: If you do choose a comfort food, enjoy a small portion mindfully.

19.8 Incorporating Relaxation into Your Routine

Relaxation should be a regular habit, just like brushing your teeth. Some ideas:

1. **Evening Wind-Down**: Set a cutoff time for work or electronic devices. Dim the lights, play calming music, or read a light book.
2. **Short Midday Breaks**: Take a walk outside after lunch or sit quietly for five minutes focusing on slow breathing.
3. **Tech-Free Hours**: Reserve certain times (like meals or the hour before bed) as phone- or TV-free.

19.9 Boundaries Around Mealtime and Work

If your day is packed, it is easy to eat meals at your desk or skip them altogether. Lack of boundaries can raise stress and harm your nutrition efforts. Strategies:

- **Dedicated Meal Times**: Give yourself a true lunch break, away from screens if possible.
- **Avoid Working While Eating**: Focus on your food. This encourages mindful eating and lets you notice hunger/fullness cues.
- **Communicate at Work**: If possible, let colleagues know you need a break. If your job is flexible, set a lunch reminder on your calendar.

19.10 Building a Support Network

Self-care and mindset improvements are easier when you have people cheering you on. Forms of support might include:

1. **Friends or Family**: Share your goals. Ask for their understanding if you decide to spend 30 minutes exercising or want to cook healthier meals.
2. **Online Groups**: Many platforms host supportive communities for women focusing on nutrition, fitness, or self-care.
3. **Professional Help**: Therapists, coaches, or nutritionists can guide you through tough challenges and keep you accountable.
4. **Local Classes or Clubs**: Joining a yoga class, walking group, or healthy-cooking workshop introduces you to people with similar interests.

19.11 Mindset Tools: Affirmations and Visualization

- **Affirmations**: Positive statements about yourself or your goals. Example: "I am capable of caring for my body" or "I choose nourishing foods that support my health." Repeating such phrases can change negative thought patterns.
- **Visualization**: Imagine yourself succeeding—cooking a healthy dinner, enjoying a workout, or feeling calm during stressful times. This mental rehearsal can increase confidence and readiness to act.

19.12 Sleep as Self-Care

Adequate sleep (7–8 hours for most adults) is a cornerstone of stress management and health:

- **Sleep-Deprivation Risks**: Increased hunger hormones, cravings for high-calorie foods, reduced immunity, and mood swings.
- **Bedtime Routine**: Turn off electronics at least 30 minutes before bed, keep the bedroom cool, and perhaps incorporate calming scents like lavender.
- **Prioritizing Rest**: Treat bedtime as non-negotiable. If necessary, set alarms to remind you to wind down.

19.13 Handling Self-Care Guilt

Some women feel guilty spending time or resources on themselves. Remember:

- **You Cannot Pour from an Empty Cup**: If you are depleted, you cannot effectively care for family or excel at work.
- **Role Modeling**: Practicing self-care sets an example for children, friends, or coworkers that looking after oneself is valuable.
- **Balance**: Self-care is not about ignoring others' needs. It is about refilling your energy so you can meet those needs better.

19.14 Balancing Perfectionism and Self-Compassion

Perfectionism can be harmful if you constantly judge yourself harshly for small missteps. A healthier approach is **self-compassion**:

- **Acknowledge Imperfection**: Everyone makes mistakes. Instead of criticizing yourself, use them as lessons.
- **Be Kind to Yourself**: Speak the same supportive words you would to a friend who is struggling.
- **Celebrate Steps**: Even partial success is progress—eating one more vegetable serving than yesterday is a win.

19.15 Adapting Self-Care to Different Life Stages

- **Younger Women (Teens to 20s)**: Balancing school, starting careers, or exploring independence. Self-care might focus on building routines (meal planning, time management) that become lifelong habits.
- **Midlife (30s to 50s)**: Juggling career advancement, parenting, or other duties. Stress can be high, so brief, effective self-care routines can help.

- **Menopause and Beyond**: Hormonal shifts or retirement may change your daily structure. Self-care at this stage can help manage symptoms, maintain mobility, and preserve mental wellness.

19.16 Journaling for Mindset and Stress Relief

Keeping a journal can be a powerful self-care tool. Options include:

1. **Food and Mood Journal**: Note what you eat, how you feel emotionally, and your energy level. Patterns may emerge, such as stress leading to overeating certain foods.
2. **Gratitude Journal**: Write 3-5 things you are grateful for each day. This can shift your mindset toward positivity.
3. **Reflection Journal**: Write about a challenge you faced and how you handled it, noticing any progress.

19.17 Creating a Self-Care Plan

Your plan might include:

1. **Daily Activities**: A short walk, a healthy breakfast, and 10 minutes of reading before bed.
2. **Weekly Treats**: A relaxing bath on Sundays, a lunch with a supportive friend, or a yoga class.
3. **Monthly Goals**: Larger tasks like scheduling a check-up with a doctor or therapist, reorganizing your kitchen, or deep-cleaning your living space.

19.18 Stress-Management Toolbox

When stress builds, having ready-to-go coping tools helps. Fill your "toolbox" with:

- **Breathing Exercises**
- **Short Guided Meditations** (many free apps exist)

- **A Favorite Music Playlist**
- **A Physical Activity Break** (dancing, walking, stretching)
- **Positive Quotes or Affirmations** in your phone or journal
- **Supportive Contact** (friend, family member, or counselor)

19.19 Overcoming Obstacles to Self-Care

Common obstacles include:

1. **Time**: A jam-packed schedule might push self-care to the bottom. Schedule small blocks—10 minutes can be enough for a calming break.
2. **Money**: Self-care is not always about expensive spas. Many tools (walking, free meditation apps) cost nothing.
3. **Feeling Undeserving**: Recognize that everyone deserves care, including you. This is a mindset shift that may take practice.
4. **External Judgment**: If others dismiss your self-care, gently explain why it is necessary. Try not to let their opinions derail you.

CHAPTER 20: BRINGING IT ALL TOGETHER AND LONG-TERM SUCCESS

20.1 Reflecting on the Journey

Throughout this book, we have explored the many aspects of women's nutrition—from the basics of macronutrients and micronutrients to the complexities of hormonal shifts, special diets, managing weight in a healthy way, and facing various life stages. We have looked at stress management, emotional eating, body image, and the role of self-care. Now, we arrive at the final chapter, where we tie all these threads together to form a long-term roadmap.

Long-term success in nutrition and well-being is more than just following rules. It is about integrating these principles into your life so they become second nature. This means forming sustainable habits, continually learning, and adapting to changes—be they hormonal, lifestyle-based, or personal preference shifts. In this concluding chapter, we will map out how to keep growing, stay motivated, and face inevitable obstacles without losing heart.

20.2 Core Principles to Remember

1. **Balance Over Extremes**
   - Strict diets can be draining and often fail. A balanced approach—enjoying a variety of whole foods, moderate treats, and portion control—tends to last longer.
   - Look at your overall eating pattern rather than obsessing over single meals.
2. **Personalization**

- Everyone's needs differ based on age, health conditions, activity level, and personal circumstances. Use the knowledge shared here as a framework but adjust as needed.
- Listen to your body. If a certain way of eating leaves you tired or moody, tweak it.

3. **Consistency**
   - Small, consistent efforts usually outweigh big, sporadic attempts. Building healthy habits into your daily or weekly routine leads to steady progress.
   - If you fall off track, just resume as soon as possible—no need for guilt or extreme measures.

4. **Mindful Eating**
   - Pay attention to hunger and fullness cues. Slow down, enjoy the taste and texture of your food, and tune in to how it makes you feel.
   - Mindfulness fosters a positive relationship with food, reducing binge-eating or emotional eating episodes.

5. **Life-Stage Adjustments**
   - Needs change over time. Pregnancy, postpartum, menopause, and older adulthood each bring unique nutritional demands. Keep learning and adapting as you grow older or your situation changes.

20.3 Building a Personalized Nutrition Plan

Step 1: Assess Your Current Status

- Look at your typical meals, snacks, and beverages. Are you getting enough protein, healthy fats, fiber, vitamins, and minerals? Are there areas of excessive sugar or saturated fat?

Step 2: Set Realistic Goals

- Use SMART goals. For example, "Increase vegetable intake by one serving at lunch each day for a month."

Step 3: Plan Meals and Snacks

- Sketch a rough weekly meal plan. Include breakfast, lunch, dinner, and maybe one or two snacks if needed.
- Aim for variety in protein sources (chicken, fish, beans, tofu), carbs (whole grains, sweet potatoes, beans), and fats (avocados, nuts, seeds, olive oil).

Step 4: Shop Smart

- Make a list before shopping to avoid impulse buys. Stick to the outer aisles (produce, meats, dairy) for whole foods, and read labels on packaged items.

Step 5: Meal Prep

- If time is tight, cook in batches or use slow-cookers/Instant Pots. Freeze extra portions so you always have a healthy option on hand.

Step 6: Evaluate and Adjust

- After a week or two, note any difficulties (e.g., not enough variety, too much work, or missing nutrients). Tweak your plan as needed.

20.4 Sustaining an Active Lifestyle

Nutrition and physical activity go hand in hand. Maintaining an active routine helps manage weight, boosts cardiovascular health, improves mental well-being, and supports muscle and bone strength. Key tips:

- **Choose Activities You Enjoy**: Could be brisk walking, dancing, yoga, biking, or team sports.
- **Vary Intensity**: Include moderate steady-state activities and occasional high-intensity intervals if you are able.

- **Incorporate Strength Training**: Building muscle increases metabolic rate and protects against age-related muscle loss. Aim for at least two sessions per week.
- **Stay Flexible**: Stretching or gentle yoga improves posture and reduces injury risk.
- **Daily Movement**: Short walks or quick stretches during work breaks add up.

20.5 Ongoing Learning and Adaptation

Stay Curious:

- Follow reputable nutrition sources, read articles from dietitians, or watch educational videos. Just filter out extreme or fad advice.
- Check if there are new findings related to women's health, hormones, or age-related nutritional needs.

Reassess Periodically:

- Every few months, review what is working. Are you meeting your protein needs? Are you satisfied with your energy levels? If not, adjust.
- Hormonal changes or shifting life demands might call for new strategies. For instance, if you transition to a desk job, you might need to adapt your activity routine.

20.6 Handling Plateaus and Changing Circumstances

You might lose some weight or gain muscle initially, then progress slows. Or maybe a new job or family event changes your schedule drastically. Stay flexible:

- **Revisit Goals**: A plateau could be a sign you need to slightly reduce or increase calories, change your exercise routine, or address stress.

- **Seek Professional Support**: Dietitians, personal trainers, or counselors can offer fresh ideas if you are stuck.
- **Celebrate Non-Scale Victories**: Notice improvements in mood, strength, or blood test results, even if the scale does not move.

20.7 Guarding Against Common Pitfalls

1. **All-or-Nothing Mindset**
   - A single slip (like a day of unhealthy eating) does not cancel months of good habits. Resume normal routines at the next meal.
2. **Comparisons with Others**
   - Each body is different. Comparing your progress or body shape to someone else can lead to frustration. Track your personal improvements instead.
3. **Over-Reliance on Supplements**
   - Supplements can fill nutritional gaps but cannot replace whole foods. Focus on real, nutrient-rich meals first.
4. **Yo-Yo Dieting**
   - Repeated cycles of extreme diets followed by weight regain stress the body. Aim for gradual, sustainable changes.
5. **Obsessing Over Calories**
   - Calorie awareness can help, but fixating on numbers can lead to stress or disordered eating. Balance is key.

20.8 Reinforcing Healthy Behaviors

Habit Loop Revisited:

- **Cue**: Tie your healthy action (e.g., taking a walk) to a specific time or event (like finishing dinner).
- **Routine**: Follow through on the walk.

- **Reward**: Enjoy the sense of relaxation or accomplishment afterward, reinforcing the behavior.

Use **accountability** methods:

- Post progress on social media if you find that motivating.
- Keep a habit tracker or calendar.
- Buddy up with a friend for meal planning or workouts.

20.9 Maintaining a Positive Relationship with Food

Develop a long-term, balanced view of food:

1. **Food is Not the Enemy**: It provides nourishment, energy, and pleasure. Avoid labeling foods as "good" or "bad." Instead, consider them "often" and "occasionally" foods.
2. **Allow Flexibility**: Savor occasional treats in moderation. This helps prevent feelings of deprivation that can fuel binge-eating.
3. **Practice Gratitude**: Recognize the privilege of having food choices. Enjoy each bite mindfully.

20.10 Adapting Through Life's Changes

- **Pregnancy/Postpartum**: Nutritional demands increase, so up your intake of protein, vitamins, and minerals. Seek a healthcare provider's guidance.
- **Menopause**: Focus on calcium, vitamin D, and maintaining muscle mass. Manage hot flashes with triggers in mind (like spicy foods or caffeine).
- **Older Adulthood**: You may need fewer overall calories but more emphasis on protein, calcium, vitamin B12, and fiber. Stay active to protect mobility.

20.11 The Role of Community and Social Support

You do not have to do this alone. Whether online or in person:

- **Join a Class**: Cooking lessons, group exercise, or healthy living workshops.
- **Online Groups/Forums**: Exchange recipes, challenges, and success stories. Make sure it is a positive space rather than one that fosters comparison or negative body image.
- **Family Involvement**: If possible, cook together or plan group activities around movement (like family hikes).

20.12 Setting New Challenges and Celebrating Achievements

Routine is great, but you may get bored. Keep things fresh:

- **Try a New Sport or Activity**: Kickboxing, dance classes, or rock climbing—something that excites you.
- **Explore Different Cuisines**: Experiment with international healthy recipes.
- **Reward System**: Treat yourself to a new workout outfit or a relaxing activity when you hit a certain goal or milestone.

20.13 Summarizing the Building Blocks of Health

1. **Balanced Nutrition**
    - Emphasize vegetables, fruits, whole grains, lean proteins, and healthy fats.
    - Limit added sugars, refined carbs, and excessive saturated or trans fats.
2. **Regular Physical Activity**
    - At least 150 minutes of moderate aerobic exercise weekly, plus muscle-strengthening activities.
    - Add flexibility and balance exercises as well.
3. **Adequate Sleep**

- Aim for 7–8 hours to support hormone regulation, mood stability, and immune function.
4. **Stress Management and Self-Care**
    - Build relaxation routines, mindful breaks, or calming hobbies.
    - Practice positive self-talk and set boundaries in relationships and work.
5. **Consistent Monitoring**
    - Check in on your mental well-being, body's signals, and any changes needed in diet or exercise.

20.14 Real-Life Success Story (Example)

Maria's Journey

- **Challenge**: Maria is a 42-year-old mother of two, juggling a full-time job. She often skipped breakfast and ate fast food at lunch. She felt exhausted, gained weight, and experienced mood swings.
- **Approach**:
    1. She began preparing overnight oats for breakfast to avoid skipping meals.
    2. At lunch, she brought a homemade salad or leftovers most days, saving time and money.
    3. She practiced deep breathing in the car before picking up her kids, reducing after-work stress.
    4. Once a week, she tried a new veggie recipe with her family.
- **Outcome**: Over six months, Maria lost some weight, but more importantly, she felt more energetic, her mood improved, and her family embraced many of the healthier dishes.

20.15 Overcoming Final Hurdles

1. **Fear of Failure**: Remember, slip-ups happen. Failure only becomes final if you stop trying.

2. **Neglecting Mental Health**: Emotional well-being is as important as food choices. Seek professional help if stress or depression are overwhelming.
3. **Too Much Pressure to Look a Certain Way**: Focus on health markers (energy, blood tests, endurance) rather than just appearance.
4. **Plateaus**: Switch up exercise, slightly adjust calorie intake, or focus on different measurable goals (like lifting heavier weights or running longer distances).

20.16 The Next Steps: Continuing Your Growth

Even after reading this book, your nutrition journey continues. Keep these suggestions in mind:

- **Stay Open to Learning**: Nutrition science evolves. Look to reliable sources (registered dietitians, peer-reviewed journals) for updates.
- **Periodically Check In**: Every few months, ask, "Am I still on track with my goals? Do they need to change?"
- **Adjust with Life**: Changing jobs, moving cities, or family changes can disrupt routines—be flexible.
- **Mentor or Help Others**: Sharing what you have learned can strengthen your own habits and build a supportive community.

20.17 Making Nutrition Enjoyable

To keep going long-term, find joy in the process:

- **Experiment in the Kitchen**: Try new herbs, spices, or cooking techniques.
- **Theme Nights**: Make healthy versions of pizza or taco nights.
- **Invite Friends to Cook Together**: Turn it into a social activity.

- **Celebrate Cultural Foods**: Traditional dishes can often be adapted to be more nutrient-dense without losing flavor or heritage.

20.18 The Power of Mindful Maintenance

Once you reach certain milestones—like stable weight or a comfortable routine—it is tempting to relax. Maintenance is a stage often overlooked, but it is crucial for preserving your results:

1. **Keep Key Habits**: If meal prepping on Sundays worked, continue doing it. If you skip it for too long, old habits might creep back.
2. **Rotate Activities**: If you walked for months, try a dance class to keep boredom away and your body challenged.
3. **Stay Attuned to Body Signals**: Weight drifting up, feeling tired, or frequent cravings might signal you need to refocus on a balanced approach again.

20.19 Gratitude for Your Body's Capabilities

Rather than fixating on flaws, acknowledge what your body does well:

- **Mobility**: The ability to walk, dance, or hug loved ones.
- **Taste and Smell**: Enjoying the flavors and aromas of nutritious meals.
- **Adaptability**: Recovering from colds, healing wounds, adjusting to new exercises.
- **Strength**: Even small progress in lifting a bit more weight or walking farther is worth celebrating.

By appreciating these capabilities, you nurture a kinder relationship with your body, making it easier to treat it well through proper nutrition and care.

20.20 Final Words and Encouragement

You have reached the end of this comprehensive guide, but your path toward optimal health and well-being is ongoing. To summarize:

1. **Self-Awareness**: Learn to listen to your body's cues, emotional triggers, and stress signals.
2. **Knowledge**: Understand nutrients, hormones, life-stage needs, and the role of emotional well-being.
3. **Practical Action**: Set SMART goals, meal plan, meal prep, choose varied exercise, manage stress, and prioritize self-care.
4. **Adaptability**: Be ready to tweak your approach as life evolves.
5. **Positivity**: Celebrate growth, practice self-compassion, and maintain a hopeful, forward-looking perspective.

Long-term success is not about never falling. It is about learning to rise each time, armed with knowledge and faith in yourself. By integrating balanced nutrition with regular movement, mindful self-care, and emotional resilience, you lay the foundation for a fulfilling and healthy life. Remember, the steps may be small at times, but each one moves you forward. Trust in the process, trust in your ability to learn, and keep striving for a future where your health supports all the other dreams and aspirations you hold.

You've got this. May the insights, strategies, and examples in this book serve as a steady guide as you continue your journey toward optimal health and well-being—both now and for many years to come.

Closing Thoughts

With these final two chapters, you now have a complete 20-chapter guide on women's nutrition, designed to be both informative and practical. By combining knowledge of nutrients, life-stage needs, emotional wellness, habit-building, and self-care, you are equipped to make lasting changes in your daily life. Remember that perfection is not the goal; consistency, curiosity, and self-compassion will pave the way for continuous growth and enduring health. Celebrate every small success, learn from setbacks, and keep moving forward on your unique path. Your body, mind, and future self will thank you.

www.ingramcontent.com/pod-product-compliance
Lightning Source LLC
LaVergne TN
LVHW012044070526
838202LV00056B/5595